Touched by Madness

Angela Thomas and Debbi Stephens

ISBN: 978-1-916732-81-0

Published by:

i2i
PUBLISHING

www.i2ipublishing.co.uk

i2i Publishing, Manchester.

CONTENTS

"No great genius has ever existed
without some touch of madness"

Aristotle

"In a mad world, only the mad are sane"

Akira Kurosawa

PREFACE

Most of us during our lifetime meet many people other than our immediate friends or families, who for some reason have a large impact on our lives. It is difficult to narrow down why some more than others seem to click with us, even though we meet by chance, arriving from very different backgrounds and places. So it was when I met my co-writer of this book. Our paths crossed by chance while we were pursuing a career in mental health nursing during the late 1970s, training at a large psychiatric hospital. We were both in pursuit of this career by default, as other factors in our respective lives had led us to this path, not being our first choice. It was a case of why not give it a try, as this just might be a job that fulfils our current needs, and if it doesn't work out, we can just move on to something else.

So in both our cases there was no deep inspiration to work in a 'caring for others' setting or any 'receiving a blinding light from above' convincing us that we had a calling or were destined to nurse those suffering with mental illness.

Now, over 40 years later, we find ourselves still very close friends, despite not spending much time together over the past 30 years, having physically moved miles apart to develop our lives with our own partners and families. Despite 10 years difference in our ages and totally different backgrounds and life experiences, there has always been a strong bond between us, and we have always been able to meet up or speak on the phone, just picking up where we left off. We are both now parents and grandparents and share so many similar views about life. It seems uncanny or even quite weird!

I, being older, retired young in my early 50s to spend time with my husband, who had experienced poor health in later life and sadly died some years ago, whereas my younger friend lives with her husband and has a fairly recently expanding family involving the arrival of young grandchildren. She continued to work in community mental health services until very recently, when, just three months shy of fifty years working in the NHS, she has finally hung up her 'hat' and joined the large ranks of 'the retired'.

Psychiatric services, as they were called in the 1970s when we started our careers, were always the 'poor relations' of the Health Service, with less money available and less importance placed on them. Probably because there was a huge stigma attached to not being able to cope or admitting to having a 'nervous breakdown'. It was best not talked about or swept under the carpet in those days. Recently, we are certainly talking much more about mental health problems, but whether we are really understanding what it all means or finding ways to help each other in this modern life is another thing.

The suggestion that my friend and I should write a book, a very honest joint memoir about how we started our careers in mental health, how things were over 40 years ago and how they changed during our careers, what we observed and experienced over the years and how we tried to help our patients or clients, seemed like something we needed to do. Many situations are relevant today, but we approached them in many different ways over the years. We both felt very excited about doing this, and the words about our memories just tumbled out of us, like we needed to put all this down in writing, to save it, or share it, or whatever? So hopefully, if you or others read these ramblings that follow, you may learn or gain some understanding about mental illness and mental health. We hope you will laugh or cry a little at some of the things that happened, or be shocked at some of the acceptable practices of the time, but maybe most importantly be 'Touched by Madness' as we both were.

We have both continued to be strongly affected by our experiences, and despite all, we both feel lucky that we had those experiences which helped us to understand much about ourselves and our fellow man, whilst forming our own very special connection and finding a really true friend in each other.

In the following chapters, we will write about our individual experiences, how we came to be in the job, commenced our training and what we experienced. Some experiences will be similar but narrated by two different authors, telling sometimes different and also similar versions from our own different perspectives.

For clarity I will be known as Angela and my co-author as Debbi. We hope to not only relate how we witnessed massive changes in the way we cared for those with a diagnosis of 'mental illness', now more commonly referred to as 'mental health problems', but also to show how humanity, people's needs, hopes and aspirations have changed very little and we all experience them. So despite changes in modern life, new fashions, expectations and new research-based treatments, we both discovered that stripping all that away to treat people with kindness, patience and respect often worked very well. Basically thinking, "If I was going through this, how would I want to be helped?"

However, we both attended school, college and various courses during the many years of our careers, and they helped in giving us a background to both physical and emotional problems, equipping us with various strategies on how to communicate and assess someone's mental state, often having to deal with disturbed or bizarre behaviour. We had to be able to adapt as new research-based care changed in both hospitals and the community. New drugs and practices meant keeping updated, which some staff struggled with, refusing to accept change, often referred to as dinosaurs in the job, and believe me, there were many of them along the way! The following chapters will hopefully tell the story of how working at 'the coal face', caring for real people experiencing problems with their mental health, influenced us both so much and touched us, so that we wanted to carry on trying to help and make a difference. We also had a lot of fun along the way too!

THE START OF THE JOURNEY FOR ANGELA

She looked at me with contempt as though I had crawled out from under a stone. "You will receive a giro in the post tomorrow as a one-off payment to tide you over. It will be deducted from your husband's unemployment benefit. That is if he qualifies for anything." I had waited for two hours in a crowded waiting room situated in the local Social Security Office to be told this. The kids had clung to me as we were accosted by the odd drunken person or unsteady guy asking for money or cigarettes. A fight broke out while we were sitting there, which was thankfully resolved by others in the crowd, leaving a very tense, unpredictable atmosphere and a feeling that something scary could erupt at any moment.

This unpredictable situation led me to say to myself, "That is the last time I will set foot in a place like this ever!" It was so stressful, humiliating and degrading. How so often, those who are desperate and find themselves with nothing are often treated by government departments designed to offer help, probably adding to their already existing problems and certainly promoting a feeling of self-loathing and shame. Walking back to our home a few miles away, because I had no money for the bus, pushing the trolley along with my three young children aged under five, from the Social Security Office in our local town, I stamped every step of the way, feeling angry and determined that from now on I would get a job somehow, provide for my children and independently stand on my own two feet. I didn't need any help, especially from any government department that made you feel the lowest of the low. Pride can sometimes be a very motivating emotion!

Early that morning, I had taken the children with me on the bus, to try to see if we were entitled to some money, as my husband had lost his job, yet despite informing the unemployment office and being promised a small amount of money to tide us over till he got a job, nothing had arrived in the post and we were 'skint'.

We didn't have a telephone, as many people didn't in those days, and trying to phone from a telephone box with three children was a nightmare. Our financial situation was getting desperate, as we had little food, and despite being up to date with all other essential bills, I knew we would soon be in trouble if no wages were coming in. I suppose I was feeling frustrated, and we were getting nowhere. My husband, despite our predicament, was still in bed when I left that morning, and I think that I had already resigned myself to the fact that he was more of an unreliable burden to me than a loving, supportive partner. Naively I thought that in those days most husbands went out to work to earn some money to provide for their wife and family, and most wives stayed at home to care for the children and do the shopping, cooking and housework. So looking for a job in my predicament was seen as quite unrealistic.

We were probably doomed from the start of our marriage, but looking back, I was too young and totally naive. I had known my husband since I was 14 years old, and despite him being seven years older than me, he was probably quite immature for his age. I was impressed by him having a car and being taken to the cinema or for a Chinese meal, but over time I became a bit bored and would have moved on, but he was difficult to shake off and pursued me with determination. I just went along with things for a quiet life and, looking back, was a quiet girl who did not have much self-confidence to demand what I really wanted.

So as time passed I was doing well at school, playing netball, and I loved horse riding, which played a very important part in my spare time. Not realising fully the implications of any physical relationship with my boyfriend, I ignorantly became pregnant at the age of sixteen, was married by the age of seventeen and had three young children by the age of twenty-one.

It was more acceptable in those days to marry young and have children young. We generally felt that we were grown up and knew what we were doing, and in some sense we were pushed more by our parents to work at a young age and take responsibility for ourselves, much more so than nowadays, where things have almost gone in the opposite direction!

I loved the children because they gave me unconditional love and brought me such happiness. Children are a joy, and although it was hard work caring for them, they kept me so busy that there wasn't much time to reflect on my life or where I was headed. I think I quite enjoyed 'playing at home making' and took pride in doing a good job if I could manage it. I never really asked for any help, as I enjoyed being independent and caring for others.

My parents tried to be supportive, but I think they felt let down that I had messed up by becoming pregnant so young and continuing to have more children quite quickly. They had never approved of my husband, yet I felt unable to tell them they were probably right all along about him. He did have various jobs, but there was a pattern of walking out or getting sacked, being misunderstood and deciding he was not going to be told what to do. So he decided he was going to start his own business, which is a tall order with a family to feed and no money. His passion was cars and motorbikes, which he loved to repair and renovate. On occasions this did prove to be a successful venture and even brought in some wages, but it was very intermittent. He was prone to behaving like a single man, like buying a drum kit or flying model aeroplanes with his mates, not his own sons, and spending money on these projects which we just didn't have.

So my resolve to find a job, support my children and be independent may have seemed like desperate measures, or was it my waking up and growing up to realise that I needed to do something to get out of this mess with no future and no hope of improving our lives? Having to always struggle financially and worry about bills arriving, or constantly looking for bargains, or doing without, was soul-destroying, and I know many people sadly live their lives this way. I was just not comfortable with this prospect and determined to make more out of my life.

I started working in a local pub three nights a week. Fortunately, my husband was happy to stay at home and babysit the children in the evenings while I worked. They were often in bed before I left for work anyway. I also worked in the local launderette for a few hours a week doing service washes, but had to take the children with me, which nobody seemed to mind in those days. These very poorly paid few hours did help supplement our income, but it was a constant struggle, with never anything to spare.

I had grown food in the garden thanks to the previous tenant who had planted apple trees and a vegetable patch. Some of the plants had reseeded and provided us with apple pies, plenty of potatoes and vegetable soups. Also the weekly Family Allowance, paid mainly to mothers of children at that time, also gave me a small income to make ends meet.

Finding a more permanent job to provide more of a regular wage was a challenge in that I would need childcare. What skills did I have? I scoured the newspapers as people did in those days to look for jobs. I had worked in offices, an industrial laboratory, a wholesale chemist in the 'ethical or prescription medication' department and in a large department store before. These were all seasonal or temporary jobs prior to my getting married and timed around the birth of my first child.

I had left grammar school at sixteen with eight O-level passes and always found academic work enjoyable. In view of my successful results, after leaving school, I had been offered a post in a local hospital laboratory with a chance to further my studies in that field, but being four months pregnant when I left school put an end to that going anywhere. So becoming a mum was my only future then, so I thought. Working full-time in any job as a mother of young children was quite unusual and frowned upon in those days. Nursery places were few and far between too. Most children stayed at home with their mothers till the age of four or five in those days until they started school.

I was sitting on the bus one day when I noticed a very large sign outside a local hospital saying, "Come and join us, we need nurses," but the magic words for me were that "we provide nursery care." That was it, nursery care, the possible answer to my predicament.

I didn't want to be a nurse, was terrified of injections, needles and medical procedures, so I thought, but I did need nursery care and a job, so I wrote a letter to the personnel officer at the hospital asking if they needed any help at all in offices or a laboratory or anything else, but that I wasn't interested in nursing and I would need two nursery places if that was possible. The reply some days later was that unfortunately they couldn't offer me any work in their offices or a laboratory but they had enclosed information about training as a nurse and that the main reason for the opening of the nursery was to encourage women with young children to start nurse training or return to their careers, as there was a shortage of qualified nurses, especially in the field of mental illness. I was disappointed with the response and remember glancing at the glossy leaflet about nurse training, but swiftly put it aside and left it for some weeks on the sideboard, thinking that was not for me.

However, one day, for a reason I can't remember, maybe feeling I was getting nowhere, I picked it up again and read it through, thinking perhaps I could give this a go, especially the part-time course initially, which would fit in with care of the children more than a full-time job.

I also had a negative view of nursing as a job and didn't feel a calling or enthusiasm for the job, especially having the fear of injections and procedures which may have involved cutting or blood, probably like most people if they are honest. Yet for me, all through childbirth on three occasions I had been very interested in all that happened, especially my two home births, during which I befriended the student midwife and thought at the time how I would have liked to have done her job.

Also, my past involvement with horses, dogs, cats and farm animals in my youth had involved caring for sick animals sometimes, from which I never shied away and always enjoyed making the animal more comfortable.

Being a mother of young children also involves much 'hands-on' activity and the cleaning up of every known bodily fluid on a regular basis.

Another negative point about nursing was championed in the snooty corridors of my old grammar school for girls when the teacher said that nursing was for 'thick' girls who had a tendency to care for others. 'Handmaidens for doctors' was quite an honourable career, but she stressed it was not for us grammar school girls.

Yet looking back in history, it was only the better class, nicely spoken girls who would be accepted for nursing. Ignorance and prejudice have a great deal to answer for. How wrong they often were with their narrow-minded and biased opinions.

After studying the information on how to train as a nurse, I decided to apply for the part-time course to become a State Enrolled Nurse. You were required to work 30 hours per week part-time as opposed to 40 hours per week full-time, and the training lasted 2 years, 6 months instead of 2 years. I completed the application forms, went for an interview and was given a place to start in four weeks at the school of nursing in early January 1974, but was invited to commence my employment at the end of December in order to attend an induction day and be measured for a uniform, then to work for one full day on the wards as a nursing assistant as a taster experience prior to going into the school of nursing to officially commence my training.

Two nursery places were made available for my three-and-a-half-year-old and 18-month-old sons, which would enable me to commence my training with some peace of mind. I would still need support from my parents and my husband at times with childcare, but I felt it could work out.

What I didn't realise at the time is that this was the start of a journey into a career that changed my life, lasting over 30 years, whilst meeting and knowing many wonderful people along the way.

Eventually the day came to attend the induction at the hospital. As I walked down the drive bordered by two large, well-manicured lawns, I thought how strange that I had lived in the area all my life, had even been born just half a mile away, yet I had never set foot in this driveway and hadn't a clue what went on inside this large set of buildings. The only thing I remember is once asking my mum as a child, "What is that place?" as we passed once again on the bus. She had replied, "Oh, it is a hospital, not an ordinary hospital but a hospital for mental patients." I had no idea what that meant but probably decided it was too vague to understand, so I never pursued it. However, I do remember all the times we rode past on the bus through all seasons; I was always impressed by the beautiful lawns and flowers, but you rarely saw any people about. It was always quiet and peaceful. Little did I know that back then most of the wards were locked and patients were just not allowed out, except with the permission of a member of staff or accompanied by a member of staff. No wonder the place always looked quiet and tidy to the outside world.

The main drive led to a lodge and bus stop from which small buses would take anyone down to The Annex, which evidently was about a mile down the road to the rear of the main hospital. I had been instructed on that first day to report to the office under the clock tower, which was past the lodge and down another drive with various buildings on either side.

Once there, I explained that I had come for the induction and was ushered to a boardroom to sit with others who were obviously there for the same purpose. We all smiled nervously and greeted each other shyly as each one arrived, making me realise that these people were all probably as new to this as me, feeling just as nervous.

I had tried to make a real effort, trying to look professional, wearing my best suit and high heels, which I hadn't worn for ages, making me feel very overdressed and uncomfortable.

Eventually an elderly, friendly man entered the room and introduced himself. He explained that we would have a brief tour of the hospital, to see some of the wards and services, then would go for lunch in the dining room. Following that, we would take a trip to the annex and then to the sewing room for those who needed uniforms. He explained that he was the 'Social Secretary' who organised social events for the inmates and introduced new staff or volunteers to the hospital in an informal way. He also informed us that he would be retiring very soon, so we may be the last group of 'inductioneers' with him. He explained that when we entered the wards, it would be nice to be friendly and natural, saying hello to any patients and trying not to just stare at people.

He also warned that we may be asked for cigarettes, and it would be advisable to say no, as the patients do have their own supply if they smoke. So the tour commenced, and I thoroughly enjoyed it, finding everything very interesting. I was amazed at the size of the place. There was a shop, a cafe for the patients and relatives, a laundry, a pharmacy, a butcher's shop, greenhouses and gardens, an industrial and occupational unit, a ballroom, a social club, male and female residences, a school of nursing and many different types of wards. It resembled a self-contained village. The annex was another small hospital in itself. The patients we met ignored us on the whole, but some came up to us to talk and were inquisitive, asking who we were, and they seemed quite 'normal' apart from wearing fairly old-fashioned, ill-fitting clothes and displaying some strange mannerisms or gaits.

I learned much later that there were lots of reasons for these facts, sadly many inflicted by long-term institutional care, up to the point that often 'long stay psychiatric patients' could be spotted in a crowd from a great distance due to these oddities. Such things like staring straight ahead, seeming to be unaware of one's surroundings, with head bent forward while shuffling along, taking small steps.

We visited the female locked ward, which housed those who, it was thought by medical staff, needed to be locked in for their own safety or the safety of others. My feelings were more of embarrassment at invading their space rather than fear of them. I was surprised to see that all patients seem to be segregated into male or female wards. They were very mixed in age groups apart from the 'Geriatric' wards, which housed those aged over 60, and so many of them were asleep in chairs. I didn't know at the time, but this was probably a great deal to do with too much tranquillisation medication and sheer boredom.

All seemed to be dressed in day clothes, and most were sitting in lounges on easy chairs or pacing up and down the ward deep in their own thoughts.

The day ended with a trip to the sewing room, where I was given some 'off-the-peg uniforms' and informed that I needed to return at a later date for any extras such as a cape or more hats, which were made of paper. We could purchase our own belts, collars and cuffs, which I later learned could become fashion items, and there was quite a competition amongst the female nurses to excel and look your best. All manner of belts, buckles, badges and fob watches were proudly worn to impress or compete with colleagues. I had several practice runs to try on the uniform at home, as the collars and cuffs were stiff and heavily starched, making it difficult to bend them or attach them to the dress. I discovered later that during a shift they rubbed on your neck and arms, causing sore red marks.

The hats were another nightmare, firstly trying to make them from a flat piece of card, then trying to place them on your head and secure them so they didn't fall off. What purpose did they serve? I don't know to this day, as they were more like a decoration with sticky-up wings rather than a head covering. I think originally nurses wore head coverings to keep their hair tidy and to prevent contamination, but these paper adornments were neither of any use nor ornament. The male nurses wore dark grey-coloured wool suits or white coats when engaging in medical procedures, so it was difficult to work out who was a doctor or a nurse. Name and title badges helped if worn!

There were a great many male nurses at the hospital, something I just hadn't considered back then, thinking that all nurses were women. From what I ascertained during some brief conversations during that day, the group of about 20 who were engaging in the induction alongside me were a mixed-age group of men and women all about to commence work at the hospital in various roles, and not all were to commence nurse training as I was.

Amongst the group, I noticed a man in the group of new staff, with longish dark hair and a beard, wearing a scruffy Afghan coat and sporting what looked like a black eye. He seemed to have a laid-back air about him as though he had seen it all before and regularly held back in corridors or outside spaces to have a smoke, whilst we eagerly followed our leader and asked questions at every opportunity. I remember thinking how scruffy and inattentive he seemed, but there was something very attractive about him. He looked like or appeared to be 'the rebel without a cause' or 'the crazy diamond' to me. What I didn't know then was that three years later he would become the love of my life, I would be in a relationship with him, would later marry him and we would spend 39 happy years together. If someone tries to tell you the future or how your life may go, you just can't always believe it.

Some people's lives are fairly predictable, but many are not, just like all those thousands of patients who, having started out much like the rest of us, found themselves in a large psychiatric hospital, sometimes for most of their lives, probably never dreaming that would be their fate.

In later chapters it will become evident that our misunderstanding of mental health and so often our inability to deal with it over the years has caused all kinds of problems for so many. The sad thing is that we are still crying out for help, with mental health issues drawing more attention than ever in our modern-day life.

The following day I arrived at Ward 4 at 9:00am to spend one day helping out as an assistant prior to a few days off over the New Year holiday and commencing my training in the school of nursing. Ward 4 was the female locked ward in the hospital, so I had actually been there yesterday during our tour of the hospital on induction. I was greeted by the charge nurse, a very pleasant and friendly young man who put me at ease and showed me around. He asked me about myself and told me a little about the ward and what their role was. We went into the dayroom, and I helped to give out cups of tea served from a large stainless steel urn. The tea went down very well, and the charge nurse dished out cigarettes to those that smoked. Then he asked me if I would like to help with bathing some of the patients. He pointed out a middle-aged woman to me, so I approached her to ask her if she would like to come for a bath. I introduced myself and asked her politely, receiving no response. I then asked her a little louder and pointed out that I would help her. Still no response until another nurse walked by and shouted, "Edith, go for a bath with that nurse now."

A bit harsh, I thought, but it worked, and Edith came with me into the bathroom. She just stood there with her arms folded and I practically had to help her with undressing and stepping into the bath. She also needed help washing, and despite my talking to her throughout the process, she never spoke once.

I found this quite strange and upsetting, so I just tried to be as kind and encouraging as I could. Why was she like this and what had happened in her life to be here in this locked ward? It became evident later during my training that some of these patients had been in the hospital for many years, had become very used to being told what to do, often quite harshly, and had lost the ability to speak or think for themselves. Quite tragic and very noticeable when you step in from the outside world on your first day.

I was then asked to help with giving medicines out and serving dinner, which was served from a large stainless steel trolley in the centre of the dining room. The charge nurse seemed to take control of this event, almost like directing a military operation. He later asked me to join him for lunch in the dining room, for which I was grateful as I didn't know anyone. The busy staff dining room was noisy, serving a good variety of hearty meals at very reasonable prices, interestingly served by many Spanish people who chatted away to each other in their own language. The whole atmosphere was friendly, and everyone seemed to know each other. There were plenty of jokes and teasing amongst the staff, who generally seemed to be a happy bunch. We ate and chatted, and over lunch I found the charge nurse so easy to talk to. I learned about his wife and family, and he about mine. Obviously liked by his staff and patients, he seemed so happy and relaxed in his job.

During the afternoon I was encouraged to look at some of the old case notes in the office to help me try to understand some of the types of problems experienced by the patients prior to my going into school to train. Doing this was a huge revelation to me. I began to realise that some of these patients had been in this hospital longer than I had been alive, even the lady called Edith whom I had assisted in the bathroom earlier. My head was full of questions.

Reading through some of the case notes, I discovered the case of a young woman on the ward who had murdered her two children and was in the hospital under section 65 of the *Mental Health Act*, meaning she could only be released with permission from the Home Office. There were some who had been in the hospital for many years, and their initial case notes were large documents written in elaborate script, showing a small passport-type photograph of them on admission when much younger. The reasons for them being admitted were often vague and unclear, using terms like 'idiocy', 'immorality' or 'insanity'. I was fascinated, with my head full of questions about their lives, wanting to get to know them and help them if I could. Basically I didn't know it then, but I was hooked, willingly setting off on an adventure to learn more about myself and help others. My first day ended with a feeling of sadness and disbelief, yet also a sort of satisfaction that maybe I could help by working here, whetting my appetite to learn more and looking forward to what was to come in the school of nursing.

THE START OF THE JOURNEY FOR DEBBI

A big city? It's not safe. You are not going there. Don't be daft! That was my parents' view and their response to me bemoaning my life. Why do you want to be a psychiatric nurse? There was no such thing as Google in those days, but I was aware of a local asylum and knew the town that it was located in embraced it somehow. I am not sure how this was apparent to me, but I recall talking about it with a team member from the hockey club when we played against them. Pretty random, that, now I think back. My dad's cousin, who was a lot younger than my dad, had told me about her work in a big psychiatric hospital in a city in the north. She was not in a clinical role, but managed the domestic services. I used her enthusiasm for her job as leverage!

I had been involved in a road accident on Christmas Eve the previous year, and I was due to go to that city's main general hospital for an appointment at the orthopaedic department. I think it was for a scan of some sort. It cannot have been that bad because I do not even remember the outcome! I had applied for nurse training locally and also to a hospital in the city; by pure coincidence, the appointment at the City Royal Hospital fell on the same day as the offer of an interview at the school of nursing. I remember telling my dad that it would be a good opportunity to have a 'pretend' interview. He took me to both appointments in his Vauxhall Viva! There is a blast from the past. What he did to occupy himself all day I do not know, but he was there for me throughout the day, sitting in the car and waiting for me somewhere, no doubt! I was to find out later that his long wait did nothing to improve his opinion of me becoming a mental health nurse. He said whilst sitting in his car he saw some "very strange-looking people". "This is not a place for my daughter." When I think back, nowadays we would not have sat in our car, situated in a car park, waiting for four hours, but would probably have sought out a place of interest in our satnav and then gone to visit it and had a wander around while waiting for a message or call to say, "I am ready." Dad didn't move, bless him.

I do not remember much about the interview at all really, but that is probably because I recall being offered the SEN training rather than RMN training, which required higher academic qualifications, as in England they said that they could not accept Welsh Language and Welsh Literature as O-level passes. I was furious and felt they really discriminated against me and the Welsh. I had worked hard for that Welsh Literature exam, and I made it quite clear to the two individuals who were interviewing me that I did not believe they could use this against me, as I knew that they had previously accepted French as a qualification from a nurse.

I was asked to leave the room and wait outside. I thought about leaving there and then, as I knew my poor dad would have been waiting in the car park, but I stayed, and guess what? Someone came out asking me to go back into the room and said they had reconsidered. I had been accepted for the nurse training course beginning in February 1978, just three months away! Can you imagine that in this day and age? There would be a meeting about a meeting, and a decision would certainly not be made there and then; it would go to an equalities committee and probably the Court of Human Rights due to discrimination against the Welsh!

Me and my big mouth, arguing about Welsh being a good qualification! I clearly remember the next question ... "Would you like to be taken to the sewing room before you leave? You can be measured for your uniforms today to save you coming all this way again just for that reason." OH NO, my dad will have a fit! The decision was made there and then; I recall the sense of relief that I was going to be employed, actually earning some money! This was unreal! ME! A nurse!

I was leaving home! My life was suddenly exciting and terrifying all at the same time. But mostly, I remember thinking I will make Mum and Dad proud. I had been such a pain in the bum since leaving school. My brothers were good as gold, athletes who were taken here, there and everywhere every weekend (and I had to go too). I remember resenting this whilst being very proud of them, but I was a huge pain in the bum! I was too busy doing sports to be concerned about my education. I also enjoyed doing things I was not supposed to as well. Going out, church youth clubs, boys, and of course pushing boundaries as always! Skirts too short, telling lies about violin lessons, hiding the damned thing in the bushes on a Thursday and just picking it up on the way home, haha! I was not the good daughter, like my brothers were the good sons!

A short walk bypassing part of the enormous walls of the hospital and seeing some strange-looking characters on the way, I was duly measured and taken back to the car park to my dad, who was totally fed up of waiting.

As I said, there were no mobile phones in those days to send a quick text; we communicated by speech and putting money in a phone box to ring a landline or letters in an envelope with a stamp on! And a lot of faith in our gut feelings, but Dad knew I was OK.

Until I got in the car, and then my bubble burst, big time! My poor dad nearly keeled over when I told him I was starting training at this big scary place, in this big city, with miles and miles of road between us and also in three months' time. "You are not…", "You can't stop me!" and on it went until I got home, and my dad, who had changed colour several times from white to red to grey, was quite pale when he told my mum of our horrendous journey home and the outcome of our day in the big city (the hospital appointment all but forgotten by now). My mum (loved and missed so much in the last years since she died) said, "She got in? Oh, WONDERFUL! It will do her the world of good to get away from here and see a bit of life." GO MUM.

You see, my mum had left a very remote part of Wales to go to Liverpool to train as a children's nurse, and that was how she met my dad. He bought her a drink, I believe, Pale Ale, when actually she wanted a Babycham, or so the story of their remarkable relationship goes… but that is another story.

The next three months were spent preparing to leave my family and friends. When I think back now, going to a big city more than 40 miles away was a really big deal! These days we pop there to do a bit of shopping or visit my wonderful friend, Angela, whom you have already met.

I could not convince my parents that I should live in the nurses' home. I was to go and live with my dad's cousin not far from the hospital. She had her own home and shared it with a friend of hers who also worked at the hospital in a non-clinical role. This was not as bad as it sounds, as I explained she was a lot younger than my dad, she was single and a good laugh. She had made a wonderful bed in the box room for me with cupboards underneath, and Mum made me a new duvet cover to take with my new duvet too! This was a very new item; at home we still used sheets and blankets and eiderdowns on all our beds. Duvets were very modern things and not easy to buy at the time. I remember the cover being different shades of pink and floral, and guess what! There was a pillowcase to match! I was so lucky.

I was to pay rent to my cousin, so for the months leading up to the big day, I worked in a local newsagent's to try to save some money to tide me over until I was paid. I remember being quite selfish during that time. I didn't think about how my mum and dad and brothers felt about me going away; I just wanted to go and start my new adventure. That was until the day dawned and I was terrified; I had many second thoughts, and I recall my dad being so falsely cheerful all the way there.

Dad went home, and all three of us sat and drank Guinness whilst we discussed and agreed our house rules, all of them pretty low-key, incorporating many trips to the pub and going to work mainly! Woohoo, this was such a grown-up world! I didn't realise at the time I was going to be exhausted and often hungry for a home-cooked meal instead of lots of cheese and bread with beer. My cousin had a very responsible job at the asylum and worked long hours, as did our other housemate. She too had a boyfriend who spent time at our house. So grown up!

BACK TO SCHOOL FOR ANGELA

Hurriedly pushing a buggy containing my two youngest children, I rushed towards the hospital nursery, constantly reassuring my kids that now they were 'big boys', they were going to a nursery to play with other children just while Mummy went to work. They knew that their eldest brother went to school and that they would go too when they were older. I had questioned myself several times that morning, thinking,"What am I doing? This is really hard work getting three children ready to go so early in the morning." Part of the anxiety was also for myself starting a new career and doubting whether I could cope with it all. Fortunately my husband had got himself a job at a local garage and had offered to drop off my eldest son at school that morning. My parents were on hand for any 'childcare filling in' duties if needed.

We were welcomed into the nursery, and my youngest son went happily toddling off once he spotted some toys, but my older child, who had been at home with me for four years, was very shy and clung on to me, so convincing him to stay was very difficult, and as I looked back whilst walking away, I saw him at the window waving with tears rolling down his cheeks. I can't describe the guilt a parent feels at a time like this, yet wiping my own tears away, I dashed to the school of nursing. In an ideal world we would be at home with our children, feeling that we had the means to live a fairly comfortable life without the stress of having to conveniently put them somewhere for hours while we work to supplement our income just to survive. However, in a modern society, influenced by material possessions, many feel that it is the norm to get back out to work, and many children now go to nursery. Now there are many combinations of childcare, such as stay-at-home dads while Mum works long hours, usually in a well-paid job, or more working from home.

Young children can definitely benefit from good nursery care, but I wonder how much they benefit from spending very long hours at nursery with rushed, stressed out and very tired parents who muddle through carrying their guilt back and forth to work. I suppose a little time at nursery and a little time with good grandparenting is the ideal recipe. We just don't know what we do to our kids emotionally when we are busy trying to run our lives and survive in our society till we see how they turn out as adults, and that can be a whole 'can of worms with mental health issues' for us all. The debate continues as to what is best for our young children. I suppose if they seem happy and healthy and are developing both physically and emotionally, then the type of care they are receiving may be the best for them.

The School of Nursing was a large detached old Victorian house situated in the grounds of the hospital, close to the local village and main road. On arrival a sign directed us to a classroom where we met our fellow students. We were advised to wear our own comfortable clothes, or 'mufti', as it was known to staff in those days. My class consisted of eleven members, eight female and three male. We were a mixed bunch of three very young girls who were 18 and had been cadets at the hospital since the age of 15 or 16, older married women, a divorced woman about my age with a young son and the men who had worked in different lines of work but decided to go for a complete change of career for various reasons.

We were encouraged to tell the whole class our name and a little information about ourselves, explaining why we had made the choice to become a nurse. We were introduced to our two main tutors, both male, who explained a little about the course, both written and practical work and final examinations. So armed with information, books, files and folders, I commenced my four weeks in school. We learned about anatomy and physiology, practical nursing skills, mental illness categories and the history of mental hospitals and then later moved on to learn about treatments and drug therapy. I drank the information in like a lost person in a desert. I loved it, learned so much about myself, started to gain some confidence and belief in myself and loved the bonds of friendship between most of us in the class.

We went to the pub together at lunchtimes, something I had never done before. In fact, I suddenly realised that since leaving school, for the past six years, I had never had any friends, just my husband and children, or been out socially anywhere apart from to my husband's sister's house for Sunday lunch occasionally, which I dreaded, because she had a 'posh' house with loads of breakable 'Capodimonte' ornaments displayed on low surfaces. I had three boisterous and inquisitive boys, so that was not a good mixture, and I was unable to relax, constantly telling them, "No, don't touch!" Basically I realised that I had probably been living a fairly sad life, being so busy and preoccupied with day-to-day survival, caring for all the family and doing nothing for myself.

Some of my classmates became close friends, confiding in each other, which made me feel as though I had some support. I know that others felt that too, as we passed through our training together. It is the case that every one of us has mental health needs, and maybe a bunch of people from all walks of life who find themselves learning and preparing how to help others, in the process gain help for themselves. Self-awareness helped a great deal in understanding how others might respond or feel when experiencing mental health problems. Whilst training there was plenty of opportunity to talk about feelings and share thoughts and experiences.

Enough of that serious stuff, because the whole experience was lots of fun too. The tutors seemed to have a great sense of humour, like tricking us into believing that in order to test a urine sample for traces of sugar in diabetes, we should dip our finger in the sample and taste whether it is sweet. Or the time when one of them was a charge nurse on the wards, and he reprimanded a patient for constantly smearing shit on the walls of the bathroom. The patient apologised and insisted he wouldn't do it again, but as he went past the nurse, he patted him affectionately on both cheeks and smeared shit on his cheeks instead.

We also had a nursing sister from the wards who came to teach us about practical nursing, from making beds to doing sterile dressings. She was very sharp, tidy, skinny and fussy, so set herself up for plenty of abuse from us. She insisted that we don't wear our skirts too short or reveal any bosom when bending over, as this could excite or offend a patient. The men in the group assured her they would keep their hemlines long! Others teased her, saying if you've got it, flaunt it.

She went on and on about wearing a good deodorant and washing your smelly bits regularly. She said that there was nothing worse than a nurse leaning over you and smelling bad. We all fantasised that she was a bit too obsessed with bodies and pheromones and would probably lean across patients a bit too often, which was quite cruel really. Something about behaving like students comes to mind, even though most of us were well past eighteen! The classroom environment and lack of responsibility encouraged this behaviour. We were getting paid and not taking life too seriously!

The younger members in the class, ex-cadets, were definitely at an advantage, as they had spent several years wandering around the hospital delivering messages, getting to know many staff, those who were in charge and how the hospital functioned. They also knew quite a good bit of gossip, which was useful when we were given our first allocation to a ward, so they filled us in on the staff, the nice ones, the not-so-nice ones and the odd ones. One of the girls was a great narrator and comedienne, maybe due to her Lancashire roots and total 'hippie' unconventional persona, but she was a joy to listen to and often had us in stitches laughing. The older women were more serious but soon cracked a smile or two when the stories were flowing. One of them was coming back to work, as her children were now older and more self-sufficient. Another was the wife of a psychiatrist at the hospital. They had married later in life, and she was desperate to have children, but she was having difficulty getting pregnant, so she had decided to do a part-time nursing course for something to occupy her. She was a bit posh and terribly naive, so we did our best to corrupt her a little. I hope we didn't go too far and cause any upset. The happy result was that she eventually left the course, having become pregnant but suffered a miscarriage, then later on had two baby boys and regularly met up with us to show off her lovely family. I was the only one in the group who was part-time and had to continue my training for a further six months, so I eventually left this group and joined another group in their final months.

It was really a paper exercise, as I didn't really learn any more but had the pleasure of gelling with another group of students, many of whom became friends too.

What I didn't realise when I started on this venture was that there were two types of training: one training as a pupil nurse on a two-year course to become a State Enrolled Nurse (SEN), which is a more practical, second-in-command nurse, or alternatively training as a student nurse on a three-year course to become a Registered Mental Nurse (RMN), who would eventually take charge of a ward or move into management. I just thought there was a part-time or full-time course. In order to take the three-year RMN course, you had to be full-time, and the course proved to be a bit more academic than the more practical SEN one, so one day during my first weeks in school, I was approached by a tutor who taught on the RMN course, asking me why I wasn't on that course due to my eight GCE passes obtained at school. I explained that I hadn't realised there were different levels of training and that I just needed a part-time job with nursery care, to be honest, but was enjoying every minute of it so far. He encouraged me to think about going full-time later on in my career, and by training another 18 months, I could become an RMN.

While we were in school, we were escorted to the laundry, the library, the pharmacy and the hospital museum, which was situated in the cellar of the school of nursing. The hospital was opened in 1851 as the County Lunatic Asylum to accommodate 500 patients and in 12 years was extended to accommodate another 560 patients, so the idea caught on quickly. Then in 1884 the Annex was built, which was a mini hospital in itself. You might ask the question, where did all these 'lunatics' suddenly come from? Well, the government was under pressure to 'do something' about all these problem people. Life in the 1850s consisted mainly of the rich and the poor. The rich were a hierarchy of male-dominated families with traditional values, supposedly high morals and 'pure' reputations to protect. So if anyone made a mistake or dared to speak out against the opinions of the day, they could find themselves in trouble, especially if they were a woman. If you don't 'toe the line', you might become an embarrassment to your husband or family and, as a result, find yourself being seen by a doctor and certified as insane!

Therefore some found themselves in private madhouses for all sorts of reasons, funded by their rich families. Things like refusing to be raped yet again by a cruel husband or becoming depressed after the birth of a child or refusing to marry someone your family had designated for you or falling in love with a lower class of person or speaking out against injustices of the day were all possible reasons why you might end up being admitted to a private madhouse. This was a great form of control, and as you can imagine, these private madhouses were strictly and often cruelly run, more attention being given to relatives' wishes rather than those of the patients.

In the case of the poor, who were extremely poor by today's standards, many of them were already living in institutions called poorhouses or workhouses, where conditions were appalling and families were broken apart. It is well documented how people dreaded ending up in the workhouse. It was the end of the line, the final straw. Many found themselves there because they lost their jobs and couldn't find work or were widowed and had children, or were evicted by a cruel landlord, or were elderly and had nobody to care for them. Losing your job could be because you wouldn't always agree to your terms of employment, which could mean working very, very long hours in cold, dirty conditions and being unwell, or maybe being physically or sexually abused by one of your bosses or managers, or having to lie, cheat or support dishonest practices against your conscience. I ask myself, are all these reasons to be locked away or to be considered a lunatic or mad? Yet many of the first residents in the new asylum came from private madhouses or poorhouses. One thing is for sure: you would certainly have had some mental health issues if you had experienced any of the above. There were no workers' unions or workers' tribunals in those days and fewer laws to aid in defending basic human rights.

The hospital buildings would have been very new and the staff newly appointed, so initially there hopefully would have been some positive ambition to make this venture a success. The institution was run in a very orderly fashion, with strict rules and discipline. Many able patients were given jobs and responsibilities, which in itself was a great thing, but without proper supervision, the practices of bullying, controlling others and just taking your own anger out on others were very common. Let us be honest: these traits of human nature remain a problem in many institutions and workplaces, but thankfully we now have more education about behaviour in the workplace, with chances to voice our opinions and even some legislation to protect us.

With hospital wards housing up to 200 patients, there was no time for much individual attention, so the weak and quiet ones probably didn't have a very good time. The rules and routine were paramount to get through each day in some kind of order. The museum in the school of nursing showed photographs of rows of perfectly made beds displaying perfect 'hospital corners'. Another ridiculous aspect of good nursing and caring for others. Who really cares if their sheet and top cover are neatly tucked in? Not only that, but all the wheels on the bed had to face in the same direction. Haha, total madness? However, I have been told by another old colleague that the reason for the wheels all being turned inwards so that they faced the same way was to prevent the nurses from tripping over them. Whoops! I even to this day admit to priding myself in doing a bloody good hospital corner when making beds – bloody idiot.

On each ward there were large roaring fires, which had to be regularly tended, and male or female attendants, as the staff were called then, had to supervise all this in addition to the cleaning of the ward. Patients were bathed in large bathrooms with no screens or privacy. Often stripped at one end by a fellow patient, dunked and scrubbed by another and dressed by yet another in ill-fitting clothes, with an attendant directing the whole process, so your weekly or fortnightly bath was probably a very humiliating experience. The poor men were shaved in a line by another fellow patient using the same razor for many till it was too blunt to scrape anything at all, when a new one would be issued by the attendant. There would probably be plenty of scars, rashes and sore faces! Welcome to the institution.

The patients who got the best life, in my opinion, were those who worked on the farm, which provided most of the food for the hospital, as they were lucky enough to have some freedom and fresh air. However, others would help with sewing, cleaning, and just about everything else that needed doing. So despite there being no time for individual needs or attention, there was a sense of safety, protection and routine in the asylum. The one big happy family feeling was generated with conditions which were probably much better than those they had experienced before being admitted there. Sayings like 'grateful for small mercies' or 'beggars can't be choosers' come to mind.

The museum provided the evidence that this is how it was and how it went on for a long time, and later on I met older staff who had seen for themselves many of these things, who told the stories that they had heard from their peers who had worked there long before them.

All that I had learned so far was just mind-blowing to me. I couldn't stop thinking about it all. I hadn't even started working on the wards yet. I couldn't get enough of it and wanted to talk about it with others. My husband was just not interested, telling me to shut up about that bloody hospital. I think he was a little jealous of my newfound colleagues, but I wanted to share with him what had happened during my day in school. Up to my starting this venture, I was there all the time for him and the children. He must have felt a little pushed out, which brings me to the fact that many working in jobs where you can talk a lot of 'shop' with your colleagues, work long or unusual hours very closely together, and deal with the raw, unusual and highly emotional side of life that the general public don't see can put a great strain on their relationships outside the job. Many police, army personnel, doctors and nurses find themselves getting divorced from a partner on 'civvy street', and many marry or remarry someone 'in the job' whom they feel understands them more. That was how it went for me eventually.

DEBBI GOES BACK TO SCHOOL

Four years later than Angela, I too was introduced to the school of nursing.

Angela has stronger memories than me of time in the school of nursing, maybe because she enjoyed the academic side of things more than me. I just knew I wanted to be a nurse; I needed to continue this learning bit to get back out there and do the job. So I did go back to school, and I recall some interesting stuff, particularly the *1959 Mental Health Act*{1} and how I made myself learn it like a parrot! To this day my understanding of mental health law comes from that time, when I learned that to use the law for the benefit of the patients would be a positive way to instigate change. We talk of this, don't we? Being vehicles of change, neither of us went into that world to do that, but change was coming, as you say, and we were just lucky that we were there at the right time. I wonder if our lives would have been different had this not been the case.

We think and talk about the changes now, and thus far we have both shared some of our memorable experiences of the time, probably memorable now because we both find it hard to believe that we were a part of some of the practices and the difficult lives those people must have led living in the institution, which was supposed to be there to care for them. Yet it would be difficult for those living in communities where they felt very vulnerable and ridiculed, or misunderstood because they displayed symptoms of mental illness. There was a great deal of care, thoughtfulness and love given behind those walls of the institution, and sadly not all the changes were for the good. Maybe we will come to that later.

The day dawned, and I got a lift to the school of nursing. I remember that it was a large old stone building with steps at the front, but it had been extended at the back, and the extension was quite modern for its time. A large room with sliding windows overlooking the grounds of the hospital, which was where I met the cohort I was to train with. I was surprised to see so many male students; I do not recall the ratio, but it was definitely more than I had anticipated. I remember an overhead projector and plastic things with writing on. It projected the word 'WELCOME' onto the wall.

A man in a dark grey suit, wearing a white doctor's coat over it, was my first contact with my future teacher in my new career. He told us that we would work hard, but be rewarded with a career like no other if we 'stuck it out'. What the heck did he mean by that? I was going to be a nurse! An Angel respected by everyone! Little did I know!

Two words… Anatomy and Physiology… I hated science and just managed to scrape through my Biology O-level. The lovely files and paper and pencil case I had in my new leather briefcase/satchel soon became scribbled on, doodled on and used for angry notes passed to others asking, "What the hell are they talking about?!" I was lost! I couldn't do this.

One morning we had sat through a lesson about medicines, and after lunch was to be the same boring pharmacist droning on about drug calculations. I know the importance of this now, but back then it was all I could do to make an effort to go back after the 15-minute break to sit through some more of that. I recall going into the classroom, and we were all talking about how boring it was going to be. I decided there and then to leave… OMG! I actually did, with another student (male), but we couldn't leave by the front door, as we would have been in big trouble, so out through the big sliding windows we went! Hilarious at the time. But remember, no mobiles to get a text telling us we really were in big trouble; we had been missed by the head tutor. Having spent the afternoon in the pub making a pint of Boddingtons bitter stretch until it was warm or at least until some older students came in and lent us some money for more. (I learned the hard way about borrowing beer money; the interest rates were extortionate!) I went home later, told my much more mature housemates about my afternoon, and they, quite rightly, gave me a good talking to. If I wanted to be a nurse, I had to knuckle down, behave and work hard.

Back to school the next day, full of worry and remorse, it was worse than I thought. "Who do you think you are?", "rude and disrespectful", "do you think you have chosen the right career?", "how are you going to apologise to the pharmacist?" Oh my God, it was so much worse than I thought. I suggested shamefaced, that I should go and apologise for my behaviour, and I was duly marched over to the pharmacy. I went in alone, and I remember my partner in crime was to go after me. Why me first? I don't remember that they probably thought I had instigated the whole thing!

The smell in the pharmacy that I was marched to was really odd. I vividly remember this: musky, sweetish, chemical, and strong. I then knew I had smelled it before. The white coat worn by my housemate smelled just like it, and she worked in the pharmacy. That is a strong memory which is not really relevant to the seriousness of that day, but strange that it came into my mind so vividly. The pharmacist was not boring at all! His job, I realised, was important, skilled and very, very technical. His staff were warm and friendly; they did not look down at me as I had expected. Haha, maybe they had never met a student nurse who had been brought to them for a bollocking before. Thankfully my housemate was nowhere to be seen, but I certainly understood her disappointment in me.

I was offered help with understanding the calculations and reassured that when I was on the wards, I would not be involved in using them for a long time to come! Whew! Thank goodness for that! All in all, those 'white-coated' smelly people in that huge echoey room full of shelves and brown bottles and labels probably saved my career. I never did tell my family what I had escaped; mind you, they probably would not have been surprised – always the rebel!

We were given a big fat book, *Anatomy and Physiology for Nurses*. It was mine to take away with me in my leather grown-up bag; it smelled new and the pages were soft, the binding all bendy. (I still enjoy smelling the pages of a brand new book!) I loved that it was mine.

I also began to love what it told me! I actually started to understand how things worked in the body and how they linked together and what happens when we become unwell or injured. When I passed my anatomy test with flying colours, I thought I was at least a senior nurse! I was a super nurse! Then we got on to the good stuff… the brain, mental illnesses and the law. I was hooked.

Learning for me had always been hard; I was just too distracted all the time. I wanted to have fun; I wanted to be the class clown.

The only thing I was good at in school was PE. I excelled at that, so I was somehow allowed to get away with it. My teachers knew they could find me in the gym or on the field if I was not in class, and the PE staff allowed this too! Sometimes I left the school, though, and went to hide with friends in the local cafe, which had a wall with a table behind it, meaning you could not be seen through the window! Therefore, Mr Twig, the truancy officer, could not see either!

I left school in 1975 and went to do a PE course in the local college, Heaven! I rarely attended the A-level subjects (politics and British constitution), but it did not matter; I was only there to do PE. After all, I only wanted to be a PE teacher. That's probably why I failed A-levels three times but got an A in my PE course. Now I am glad that nobody explained to me that I could not go to teacher training college with only a PE A-level; if they had, I probably would not be where I am now.

But this, nurse education, was different; I wanted to learn, and it all just fell into place really. I started spending time lying on my bed actually reading and testing myself, and my housemates helped too. We still drank beer, though! My cousin worked in a pub some evenings, and I would go and sit by the bar while she worked, and it was there I learned how to read the horses. All those numbers in the newspapers on the racing page, they mean how the horse has done in previous races.

I used to go down the road to put bets on for the men who sat by the bar and who didn't want to get wet in the rain! BEER

MONEY - easy to earn then. There is another vivid memory! The hiss, shhhh, of the beer as it came out into the glass when she pulled the lever of the pump. It was frothy and smelled delicious.

It was there I learned to pull a proper pint when it was busy. It had to have a perfect head on it too, otherwise big trouble from the betting men. It was all men too, heavy with cigarette smoke and quiet, thoughtful pondering and scribbling on betting slips with little, tiny pencils they kept behind their ears. Now and then there would be roars of laughter. Jokes I never really understood. A man's world!

When I had finally realised that I had a responsibility to either pass or fail, to become a psychiatric nurse or not, I realised I had suddenly grown up! I did want desperately to make my family proud, and I wanted to know more about what went on behind those huge high walls at the hospital and what had happened to the people I saw wandering about the grounds, mostly wearing ill-fitting clothes, with strange walks and mannerisms and usually in a world that was not involving others around them, me especially.

I have to be totally honest here; I was actually paid a salary too! I had a month's wage of £164! I was so happy; I had never had so much money! I paid my rent and went shopping! I bought an Adidas tracksuit for each of my brothers (ugh, they were dark green with yellow stripes! At the top of the range for the time). I bought gifts for Mum and Dad too, though I do not remember what, and I got a train home for two days before I was to start on my first ward. I had never been on a train either. Gosh, I was so grown up! Dad picked me up from the station, and I don't think I stopped talking for the whole weekend! Dad took me back to the big city after our few days together. He was so worried; he didn't want me to go back. He really could not understand why I had chosen this career. Why couldn't I be a 'proper nurse'? But Mum would calm him down and convince him that I was sure! I was certain of my future.

THE FIRST WARD EXPERIENCE FOR ANGELA

Following the completion of four weeks' training in school, we were each allocated to different wards in the hospital where individuals were first admitted for assessment and/or treatment from their home, following a change in their behaviour or visit to their family doctor or, sadly, via the police suspecting they were experiencing a mental breakdown of some sort. We would spend eight weeks of experience on one of these wards, then go back into school for four weeks to consolidate our experiences and prepare for new ones.

I suppose I could consider myself lucky because I was sent to a fairly newly opened, detached, modern, purpose-built unit for mixed-gender acute admission patients, seen as one of the most modern, groundbreaking units at the time. It made sense to be there at the start of someone's mental health problem, to learn how they initially presented and what treatments could be offered. This new unit was the pride and joy of the two consultant psychiatrists in charge of care, and they were seen in the field as quite progressive then, one of them even publishing books and lecturing in the USA about psychiatric illnesses and treatment.

I wasn't aware of that back then, just that I had to arrive at 8:00am and report to the nursing office. Dressed in my brand new stiff uniform, wearing a white hat with wings (?) and a navy wool cape lined with bright red, not dissimilar to something Dracula would wear, I arrived at the office, forced a smile and said, "Hello." The young woman behind the desk wearing jeans and a scruffy sweatshirt raised her head, flicking her long fringe back, and said, "Hello, bloody hell, what have you come as?" I told her my name and that I was reporting for my first shift, and she informed me that she was the sister on the ward. What I didn't know was that she encouraged her staff not to wear a uniform, as it often created a barrier between staff and patients in her opinion. When she discovered that I couldn't just nip back to the nurses' home to get changed, she muttered that perhaps they could hide me away for the rest of my shift, and tomorrow could I come dressed as a normal person. That was a bad start, I thought, but she was quite a rude, arrogant bitch in my opinion, which I obviously kept to myself as she was the boss!

Eventually, another nurse was summoned and asked to show me around the unit. There was a lounge, kitchen and dining room, several corridors which led to a male dormitory on one side and a female dormitory down the opposite corridor. There were showers, baths, a clinic room, a conference room and various offices for interviewing patients or teaching staff, etc. I was made aware of various safety measures, including fire exits and doors that could be unlocked from both sides if someone locked themselves in and was considered at risk. We entered the lounge, or day room, and we sat chatting with some of the patients. Some seemed to be perfectly well to me, and others seemed a bit withdrawn, not interested in their surroundings.

One young man whom I shall never forget reminded me of Buddy Holly in appearance. He raced about the place smoking, in and out of rooms, often muttering to himself, yet if he passed you by, for instance, in the corridor, he would always say, "Are ye alright?" without even looking up. It was explained to me that he suffered from schizophrenia and his diabetes was very unstable because he didn't look after himself properly at home. If there were any cups of tea available, we would always know where he had been, as there was always a trail of slopped tea on the floor behind him. Sadly, despite medication, he seemed very agitated, tormented by voices to whom he responded, and was unable to sit and chat or even sit down to eat. I also learned that instability in diabetes can severely affect one's mood too.

As a result, his quick bite of food on passing wasn't helpful to stabilising his diabetes. He was always very pleasant and polite but didn't stop to chat with anyone. I was horrified when I came back on duty one day to discover that he had hanged himself in the toilets one evening, but the worst bit was that he stood on a chair, tied his noose onto a toilet cubicle frame bar, and when another male patient came by, he asked him to "move the chair over there, mate," which the other patient did, not realising what this meant, and didn't tell anyone. Later a nurse found him while routinely checking round the ward, but it was far too late to revive him. For me this was a rude awakening to the seriousness of some severe mental health problems, never to be forgotten.

I could see that his death had a large impact on the staff. Despite their jokes and bravado, they were devastated and felt they had let him down. There was much discussion in the nursing office as people came and went between all ranks of staff about what happened, and this was definitely their way of trying to deal with it. Talking and sharing can be very helpful. The office was always a hub of people coming and going: social workers, doctors, and new staff coming on duty or the handover after a shift to new staff coming on duty, explaining what had happened up to date. Oh boy, did things happen every day, and it felt like an exciting challenge each day coming to work. I met and became familiar with most of the staff on the ward, who were friendly and helpful. The charge nurse, a very cool and relaxed tall man who was loved by everyone, helped me give my first injection in my first week, on my first ward, to a real patient. Little did he know that I was terrified of needles and had already decided secretly that if I have to give an injection, I will just get my coat on, go home and give up the nurse training bit. But the whole thing was sprung on me at the last minute with no time to make excuses, and I daren't say, "Well, I am too scared to give an injection – let me get out of here."

The patient was to have a deep intramuscular depot injection, which were often given in those days on a weekly, fortnightly or monthly basis in large clinics all over the community, mainly to help control disturbing symptoms of a psychotic illness.

The drug was a slowly released thick oily substance which hopefully protected the patient until their next dose. Seen as a major advance in the treatment of severe mental health problems, these drugs were discovered in the 1950s. This particular man was having his depot injection before he was discharged home today, and he seemed to be very well. The charge nurse drew up the injection, explaining to me how to do it and that the liquid was very thick and oily, so it was necessary to take your time and administer it slowly. He showed me how to dispel any air bubbles and why, then asked the man to drop his trousers, which took me by surprise. He explained that the injection needed to be given deep into a large muscle, and the outer upper quadrant of the buttock was usually the best site on the body. Having drawn an imaginary cross on the man's now bare buttock, he pointed out the upper outer quadrant, put the syringe in my shaking hand, quickly asking the man if he minded if I gave the injection as a student and guided my hand into a dart-like position, stabbing the buttock quickly and deeply at 90 degrees to the body, to my horror, and then let go, telling me to slowly draw back the plunger a little to check for any blood, and if there was none, slowly push in the fluid, which I did. I must have stood there shocked and motionless, because he brought me to my senses by saying, "Take the needle out then; this guy is getting his arse cold." He asked the patient how it was, and he replied, "All right, nurse." I could have kissed them both, as I was so chuffed that I had actually done an injection, which I didn't, of course, as it would not have been very appropriate when one of them had his trousers down! I never looked back after that, and many, many years later I met that same patient in a community clinic and gave him his injection. I was relieved to see him still alive and well.

The staff taught me so many things on that ward, not so much about physical practical care, as the patients generally looked after themselves. However, on admission all patients were thoroughly assessed both mentally and physically, because many physical illnesses can present with all sorts of mental symptoms too.

A proper assessment could be a long process when someone was upset, frightened or very withdrawn and depressed. The admission process hoped to gently gain the patient's confidence if possible, gathering as much information as possible in order to discover what the problem was or how they were feeling. This would be initiated by a nurse. Sometimes the patient was too disturbed to talk, so any friends or relatives might give their version of events. It was often about waiting until the patient was well enough to communicate, and this could take some time. Drugs were offered to help calm agitation. However, if someone was admitted under a section of the *Mental Health Act* and considered to be a danger to themselves or to others, emergency medication could sometimes be given without the patient's consent. This didn't happen very often, but yes, I have plunged a needle into a very unhappy young man being restrained by four staff and threatening to "kill all of us fucking bastards" as we prevented him from throwing chairs around the ward and smashing the place up. On admission all new patients were seen by the ward doctor, given a full physical and mental state examination and prescribed some treatment, which could be medication, occupational therapy, supportive talking therapy or relaxation therapy, while observation and assessment continued depending on what the problem seemed to be.

A very manic Italian woman who was as wide as she was tall was admitted and certainly created some mayhem. She was loud and aggressive, yet at other times very funny and happy, but totally unrealistic. It was amazing to see her gradually change to a sleepy, quiet person with medication and eventually go home in a stable, calm mood. She was a regular on the ward evidently, as many were. The staff knew many of the patients and their relatives well, especially those who came back into hospital from time to time following a relapse.

This often happened if they stopped taking their medication because they felt so well or something in life had caused them unexpected stress. I also witnessed some people being admitted to the unit who appeared mentally disturbed, but after investigation their problem was of a physical nature, such as an infection. Most patients eventually went home well, but a few stayed in that unit for a long time for a number of reasons.

Working on the unit was fun, as again we formed friendships with colleagues and patients. We escorted them to X-ray for various treatments, played games with them, and went for walks, all the while talking and trying to build up a rapport and help them feel comfortable enough to share their worries and feelings. This being the main essence of mental health nursing, I suppose. All most of us want in life is to feel there is someone there for us who can listen, not judge and allow us to make our own decisions moving forward with support. Sadly, even nowadays many suffer from mental health problems and feel they don't have anyone like that who is there for them.

Another form of treatment often prescribed for those who may be severely depressed or psychotic and for whom nothing seemed to be helping was ECT, electroconvulsive therapy. This was performed one morning per week in another ward at the hospital, and as students we would escort our patients there, assist with the treatment and escort our patients back to our ward. This treatment involved passing a small electric shock through the brain by the use of electrodes placed on either side of the head. The patient was given a small dose of anaesthetic and a muscle relaxant before. The whole thing only lasted a few minutes, and many patients seemed to improve over the weeks, but just after the treatment they were very sleepy, and many lost their short-term memory for a little while. The scientific evidence behind the treatment, then, as we were told, simply is that the electric shock induced a mild epileptic seizure in the patient's brain, and very few people who experienced epilepsy had any severe depression or psychosis. Most patients were terrified of the treatment, understandably, but all said they didn't feel anything or forgot if they did. As nurses we witnessed the patients lying relaxed and asleep, then as the shock was administered, they would shake slightly, and we would hold them wrapped in a blanket to stop them banging or hurting themselves. I have to admit I was alarmed when I first witnessed it but saw for myself several patients become well after a few treatments. Was it the ECT or was it something else that caused the improvement?

I don't think ECT is used nowadays, or maybe very rarely. In the days previous to my training, we were told it was given 'neat' to patients without the anaesthetic or relaxant, which must have been terrifying. As with all types of health treatment, research and new knowledge have changed many practices, hopefully for the better.

The weekly ward round, which was held in a large comfortable sitting room each week with the whole multidisciplinary team sitting in a semicircle, was overseen by 'God' – no, sorry, I mean the consultant psychiatrist. It felt like God was presiding sometimes and was quite an eye-opener to me. Being at the bottom of the pecking order, it was my job to fetch the patients to the room to be seen as their case came up for discussion. I had in my mind that a psychiatrist chatted with you for hours while you lay on a comfortable couch expressing your innermost feelings, but this was something totally different. I must have actually been thinking of a psychoanalyst who may use the couch, whereas the psychiatrist was more of a medical man, prescribing drugs and treatments, requesting investigations and generally being the expert and calling the shots.

Once the team had discussed the patient's progress, the patient was brought into the room and asked about his or her view of their progress by the consultant. This was often a very different story, as some couldn't see that things were better or they were not being exactly truthful. Some were begging to go home, which I thought was quite healthy, whereas some wanted to stay and begged not to be discharged, obviously because what was outside must have been worse for them than being on a psychiatric ward. There were often tears or anger, and a few stormed out, slamming the door. It was a time when the consultant would challenge them or maybe say what they didn't want to hear. I know I felt that if I had been in the patient's shoes, I would have been terrified sitting in front of this panel of experts, being asked quite personal questions, when your confidence was already at rock bottom. All I can say is that it sorted the 'wheat from the chaff', as there were also a minority of patients who were either being manipulative, hiding from the law or not being totally truthful, and they were easily exposed by a united team of staff who shared their observations over a period of time. It was hard to understand why anyone would want to stay in a psychiatric ward when they didn't need to be there and there was little wrong with them, but by that very fact, it revealed that they had problems of some sort. Maybe they couldn't cope in the outside world very well, felt lonely or felt they had nothing to return to. They could have been afraid of something or someone or quite liked being looked after in this one big happy family with its routine, warmth, regular food, someone to clean up for you and someone to tell you what to do next. It is a common fact that some will deliberately get themselves admitted to a hospital or even prison to feel safer.

The team would discuss each patient's progress, and treatment might be changed, continued or discontinued by the consultant, and he or she would explain this and any reasons for it to each patient as they came in.

On this ward I mentioned previously that some stayed there a long time, and most of those were young, ranging from 16 to 20 years old. They seemed to have little wrong with them, but it was explained that they had personality problems, which often displayed themselves in moody, destructive or violent behaviour.

There was quite a great deal of self-harming, and this seemed to be infectious. If one slashed their wrist, then they all did over the next few days. So I learned how to suture and dress wounds. Then we had the knife-swallowing episodes, which entailed going to casualty at the main general hospital with various individuals to have surgery. It became a joke that we would request they be fitted with a zip next time, as swallowing anything was the 'self-harm craze' of the day. It was seen as attention-seeking and manipulative behaviour, which it probably was, but nobody seemed to get to the bottom of why. There was definitely a copycat element, but young, misguided and unloved sprang to mind with them all. There didn't seem to be any stable or supportive role models at home for them. They seemed to be the 'amusement' of one of the consultants who kept them in hospital for many months or even years, trying all kinds of medication, seeing himself as a specialist in this field. Some did go home eventually with a great deal of social work support; others succeeded in killing themselves, and one young man ended up in a locked ward because he kicked against any authority and eventually ended up in prison after brutally murdering someone. Having a 'personality disorder' was often given as a diagnosis for those who couldn't cope, who messed up in life, abused drugs and alcohol, or became violent, or had a history of breaking the law. I hate to say it, but most of the population could fall into that category at some time in their lives. In a more tolerant and understanding society, maybe we do not judge now as we did in those days, but somehow I don't believe we have got it right yet. I am still an advocate of children needing love and support but having boundaries too, so that they grow up knowing right from wrong and how to share and care for others, in addition to themselves. Sadly, sometimes the chemical and physical mix in one's brain is just not right, leading to severe mental health problems despite all the love and care in the world. It is often impossible to know why individuals are struggling in life sometimes, but learning strategies on how to deal with one's emotions and how to move forward in a positive way can often be a helpful start.

One patient on the unit was a middle-aged, well-spoken, quiet and polite man who didn't display any obvious disturbing symptoms, so I studied his case notes to discover that he was admitted from prison after strangling and killing his wife at home. He had done this while being severely depressed and immediately afterwards, when he realised what he had done, tried to take his own life but didn't succeed. As a result, he was treated in hospital for his self-inflicted injuries, sent to prison on remand and later admitted to our unit for treatment on a section 65 of the *1959 Mental Health Act*{1} meaning he could only be discharged with permission from the home office. I decided to do my case study on him and tried to build up a rapport with him, but he didn't share much. He had been a bank manager and had become severely depressed, not sleeping, worrying and feeling very anxious, probably over a long period of time. Sadly nobody spotted the deterioration in his mood, and when his wife was one day "having a go at him to snap out of it", he did snap but with tragic consequences. He was so full of guilt and shame and was a high suicide risk. He had two young adult children who were obviously trying to come to terms with the fact that their father had murdered their mother. It was a very sad situation, which drove home to me the seriousness of severe depression if ignored.

As you can imagine, when my fellow students and I returned to school, we had plenty to talk about, sharing our experiences from our time spent on our various admission wards.

DEBBI'S FIRST WARD EXPERIENCE

Our shift started at 7:00am. My pale blue uniform was stiff; it had big square pockets and poppers to fasten up the front. I wore a stiff paper/cardboard hat held on with hair grips and a cape made of very itchy wool; it was navy blue and red inside, and the straps were red and crossed over like an X across my chest. It was warm but not what I would call 'cosy'! It was so itchy around my neck that I couldn't wait to take it off. That cape became a Superman cape many years later for our children - they complained that it was still itchy then!

I met with several other student nurses in our pristine uniforms under the clock tower by the grand main entrance; it was 06:30am. There were qualified staff, their uniforms much washed and softer, even faded in colour. The male nurses were wearing overcoats of different styles and colours, one or two of them having their white coats under their arms. They took very little notice of us really, as they seemed busy catching up with each other's news or just shuffling on the spot waiting to start another 12-hour shift. Also smoking - everybody seemed to smoke! Usually opening packets of tobacco and rolling them quickly and deftly. I remember thinking doing 12 hours would mean not actually being in daylight for possibly five days in the winter! I thought that could not be true, so I dismissed it. I was later to realise that it really was true, and if you did overtime, well then, it was strange to see the sun during the winter months.

As I got off the minibus which took us from the main hospital down to The Annex (which was another mini hospital about a mile away in the grounds of this big rambling place). I recall trees, lots of trees, overgrown bushes and shrubs and birds tweeting everywhere. I was anxious, of course, but excitement was a stronger emotion.

I made my way to the ward I had been allocated and was welcomed by a group of staff who all met in the office to have 'a brew' and handover from the night staff. The atmosphere was relaxed; most of us stood, as there were not enough chairs. The ward was old and huge; faded, once red, lined velvet curtains hung from enormous windows which looked out over the many trees around the annex.

I recall three ladies wandering about in nighties; they were split up the back, and I could see their bums. These ladies did not interact with the staff, and the staff largely ignored them until we had been told about any issues during the night and the night staff left to go home to bed.

I was allocated to a friendly middle-aged auxiliary nurse (I shall call her Mo for now), who wore a green uniform which was faded, giving the impression she had been working in this place a long time. I recall a very broad accent; she emphasised her 'R's' and chatted warmly, not just to me, but when we entered the dormitories, she called out, "Morning, ladies! Me again today!" and "Look, we have a new girl! C'mon, up ya get!" She clapped her hands, and the ladies got up. They started to wander in their bum-flashing nighties towards the bathroom. I remember thinking that the skin on their bums looked loose and wrinkly, a bit like crumpled-up tissue paper. More staff were creating a line like a queue to use the bathroom. (More about the bathroom later).

The beds were approximately 4-5 feet apart, and the room held about 20 beds. They were heavy metal frames with sheets and cotton blankets and a 'counterpane' (a kind of heavier decorated cover/bedspread but not as warm as today's duvet or even an eiderdown) on the top. Everything looked so 'poor'; the blankets were washed out, and the counterpanes a past effort to provide some brightness, maybe? Certainly not warmth; they were faded, and some of them had damaged hems and fraying edges. We had two metal trolleys, one with two laundry bags attached on big hooks; one bag was red and the other white. One for soiled and one for clean linen. The other trolley had clean sheets, folded, ironed and strangely heavy. Mo told me that we need to check the beds and do not put clean sheets on unless they have been turned. This meant bottom and top sheets turned head to toe; you could tell if they had because they were so firmly ironed it was obvious that the bottom (feet end) were not creased!

I am still not sure if Mo intended what followed to be a deliberate initiation attempt or not, but I went to the first bed as directed, and when I lifted the pillow (only one), underneath was a large cold 'turd' (sorry, I don't know how else to describe it really) and a set of dentures! What the hell?! I was horrified, but Mo just shrugged and told me to go and get some "bog roll and chuck it in a toilet, and on the way back get a false teeth pot holder from the sluice".

I did as I was told and passed six toilets with no doors, all with ladies sitting on them, until I found an empty one to gather some toilet roll before another lady went in. There was a lot of noise, shouting, laughing, calling out of names, squealing, and the first time I had heard a woman scream out, "Leave me alone, you fucking bitch." It was echoey in the 'bathing area'. Although I was no angel, the swearing shocked me; I had never heard it used so profusely. I remember my older brother throwing my younger brother against a wall at home because he "used the F word"! And here I was at work, with the words pouring out of people's mouths as if it were quite normal! ... well, it was. I soon learned that if you could not carry fags in your pocket or swear like a trooper, you would not make it.

When I returned with loo roll and a pot, Mo had taken the case off the pillow and replaced it with a clean one. Thank God for that! I thought she would turn it over or something! I picked up the cold turd in lots of toilet paper and took it to the bathing area, where another nurse helping a lady vacate a toilet said, "Chuck it in there, Chuck," and carried on. I quickly washed my hands under a tap that was left running with hot water. There was no soap or towel, but I guessed better than nothing. I wiped my hands on my uniform and went back to making beds. Mo was singing to herself and asked me if I was "ok, Chuck?" Erm... "Yes," was my reply, (I will not be caught out by tricks, haha.) I learned how to make a proper bed that day; I learned how to decide which deserved clean linen and which didn't. I still don't understand why the beds had to be made in such a way that nobody can get in them without a struggle, and they certainly barely moved all night! Hospital corners! The beds must have been like coffins.

Whilst discussing with other staff later, I learned that the lady who kept her own shit and her teeth under her pillow probably did so because she didn't actually have any personal possessions at all. In fact not one of the patients did, and it was not uncommon to find this. As I remember this, I think to myself, "How on earth can that have happened?" Imagine a life with nothing. Nothing at all, except your own false teeth. Think about it, if you go into a hospital today, at least you have a bedside locker and maybe a small wardrobe to put your clothes/nightwear in. You will have your own toiletries and maybe an iPad or a book, oh, and probably a phone! If you are unfortunate enough not to have these items, as some homeless people or individuals with an enduring mental illness are, you will be given items, but they will be yours, not shared with others on the ward.

These people lived sometimes for many, many years in these asylums, and they did not own a thing! The clothes they were dressed in were not theirs. They did not choose what food to eat and when; they had no choice about when to go to bed or when to get up or what to watch on TV.

Do you know what I saw one day, which I have never forgotten? A lady had been knitting a bright red square, not a scarf or something to call her own, just a square. It was called occupational therapy, as it was back in the day! The wool was finished, and the square was taken from her with lots of "well done" and "you finished it, well done"... It was then taken from her, unravelled and rewound into a big, fat red ball, and then given to another lady, as it was "her turn now".

That just made me so sad.

From then on I vowed I would ask all my knitting relatives to save their wool scraps, and lady number 1 would make herself a scarf to keep. Little did I know that supervising the use of dangerous knitting needles would be so time-consuming! If lady number 1 wanted to make a scarf (which also had to be supervised and locked in a cupboard with the fags), then I would have to do it. I did it over the 12 weeks I was there, and she did complete a very colourful scarf, and we had permission to leave the ward together for a five-minute stroll in the grounds to try it out! :) Happy day! I often think of that lady and hope she was able to wear that scarf many times. (It was always locked away, though, as it was a ligature risk, but it was hers). She was a quiet, almost serene lady; she was tall, polite, always moved away from any trouble on the ward, spoke little and smiled less.

However, despite her mouth not smiling, her eyes did occasionally, and the squeeze of my arm from her strong hand as we walked out that day told me she was happy, even if it was short-lived. I was so pleased that I had been allowed to do this. I did not face any criticism from the long-serving staff; in fact, some of them helped by supervising on my days off… One nursing assistant even brought in a ball of bright pink wool.

This experience gave me a good grounding to develop my attitude of not conforming, and if you feel it right to challenge something that really does not feel right, then you should challenge, whatever the outcome.

Maybe that is why after all this time, I truly believe that if you ask yourself the question, "If this goes wrong and something awful happens, could I stand up in court and tell a coroner that I did it with the very best intentions and that I had considered counterarguments but still carried on…?" If the answer is yes, then do it. I still firmly believe in the philosophy of recovery and always have. Recovery today means something very different, and maybe if I get to that point I will explain myself; however, then it was more about giving the opportunity for something nice to happen in an individual's day. The actual future existed only from rising to bedtime; there was no next week, month or year. It was a life without dreams and aspirations for those patients.

I did my first case study on lady number 1. I was allowed into the dark, damp, smelly bowels of the administration block of the hospital to find her old case notes. I was so shocked I wept! How could I be with her again? I was overwhelmed with sadness and uncertainty.

The case notes were big, almost like a broadsheet newspaper, and there was a small photo of a much younger-looking lady number 1; she had proper hair (not thin and wispy), she had flesh on her face (not gaunt features with thin yellow skin), the writing was fancy and in proper ink (not ballpoint pen), she had lived in a nice part of the world and had a husband and children. She had had a life. However, this lady number 1 had murdered her twin babies.

I didn't want to do that case study, but to be honest I had spent so much time supervising the damned knitting I didn't have time to choose another patient! So I did it, and I passed my first real piece of academic work that was going to turn me into a nurse! But it also began to help me understand the dreadful illness now known as postpartum psychosis, which thankfully can be successfully treated today.

Providing it is recognised early, medication is provided and compassionate staff are there to help throughout the difficult times. One of many sad things I learned in the early days is that the condition was misunderstood, and many women did awful things to their babies, children or themselves, often under the influence of terrifying hallucinations or delusions, and were severely punished or mistreated. Their partners and relatives also lacked any education or knowledge about the condition, so often rejected their suffering relative and had them incarcerated in a mental hospital forever.

Back to owning nothing, a concept hard to believe these days, as I said, but on the ward there were two other ladies who did own something... One glass eye each, having lost an eye, which was probably quite common in the 1920s-1930s, who knows? Anyway… I hated cutting nails, fingernails sure, but toenails made me heave, especially as all the feet had not had the benefit of well-fitting shoes, foot spas and nail painting! Oh my lord, it was a thankless job… So I swapped… I did glass eye cleaning, which, strangely, lots of the other nurses could not do. It was easy… just press under the eye, and out it came, bit of a wash, and hey presto, done! The socket is cleaned, and it is placed back in. Where was I? Oh yes, possessions… I confess I put the wrong eye in the wrong socket one day, so both ladies had one blue and one brown eye all day. So sorry, ladies. One or two members of staff noticed, but not Sister, who would have given me hell! Each lady had their own eyes back the next day, and I learned another valuable lesson… take your time, don't rush, and check what you have done!!!

I have to say that owning up would have been futile anyway; things were done in such routines on the ward. The thought of getting those two ladies into the clinic area (such as it was) would have caused untold problems. Routines had to be kept without question.

When I think back now, 12-hour shifts from 7:00am to 7:00pm sound very long, but do you know, the days just flew by! I was much younger then and full of energy and enthusiasm. I was desperate to learn and do a good job. There were, however, two categories of staff to learn from, and I had to learn very quickly how to avoid or deal with the group whose practices sometimes bordered on cruelty. On the whole they were in the minority, thank goodness, but they were actually strong and influential. I am not sure that they ever really considered that what they were doing was wrong in any way, as these were practices which had been embedded in time and should not be changed just because some 'jumped up' student nurse thought it was wrong.

One example which springs to mind stays with me because I could not understand how the kinder, more caring staff allowed it to continue. Breakfast was served from a big steel trolley. There were three huge, battered teapots made of aluminium (I know this because I don't like the feel of it; to me it was like nails scraping down a blackboard) which contained tea with the milk and the sugar already in (tough if you prefer your drink without!). There was a tray with sausages and bacon, or sometimes one or the other, and also a large pan of porridge. Oh, and there was toast. Well, it was toast when it left the kitchens, but by the time the van arrived with it from the main hospital, it was just floppy bread, really.

Three or four of the ladies found it difficult to sit still; they paced up and down the ward all day, muttering to themselves, hand wringing and moving their mouths constantly; their poor jaws must have ached so much. These were side effects of the medication they were given, but I will come to that.

Because they found it difficult to stay still, they were placed at one table in the corner at meal times in 'geriatric chairs'. These chairs were heavy, with small wheels and a table in the front, a bit like a giant child's highchair really. I noticed that although the table areas were clean, the wheels and metal bits were often dirty with old dried-on food. Ugh, and it was to these dirty metal bits we had to tie the ladies' legs with stockings (soft so as not to hurt them!), a very common mealtime practice. One male nurse would give porridge to three ladies and toast to another; no choices offered, I am afraid, and I believe to this day that he wanted the sausages for himself to eat on his break.

One lady with the toast would become angry and shout at the ladies with their porridge, then one day she threw a plate at the lady opposite and badly cut her head. It was awful to see. I observed this frustration about not getting porridge a few times, but in the morning, as everyone was so busy getting the damned routines completed, that same male nurse seemed to continue to not offer choices and hide food away. The poor frustrated lady would be punished for her aggressive behaviour. 'Punishment' may be a strong word; however, it was punishment that particular day when she threw the plate, because she was put in a 'policy room' (a bare room with a mattress on the floor) and was given enough medication to flatten a horse.

I recall her screams and anguish on her poor face as she was dribbling and spitting. He knew she would react; it was almost like a sport. I hated it.

Suffice to say when he wasn't there she had porridge and toast; no one was hurt, but they were still tied to the chairs. "It's for their own good"; apparently they wouldn't have a good diet if they were allowed to pace around. Sadly their legs still jiggled about and knocked at the tables above their legs. You would be right to ask why it was not challenged. I was in part, without discussing it, too afraid to highlight it for fear of recrimination, but we did our best to manipulate the breakfast serving, though.

One day I was a bit blatant and said I would serve the tied-up ladies, and he couldn't really challenge me, but I paid for that… as when the shift was over he deliberately made sure I couldn't get on the first bus back up to the main hospital, and I can still see his horrible smirking face looking me straight in the eyes as the bus departed… Another 20-minute wait for me! I guess that was his futile attempt to tell me not to mess with him. I have no idea how his white coat got iodine all over it one day or how his sausages hidden in the sluice ended up in the bin! Haha, a small thing, but it made me feel a bit better!

That man had worked at the hospital for many, many years, long before the days of student nurses arriving on the wards; he was probably called an attendant back in the day, and I have to say I was convinced that if he was asked to be more compassionate, the poor patients would have suffered more in private.

Thankfully the likes of him were being replaced with much kinder people as these cruel individuals were dying off, or at least retiring! It was a very precarious situation; maybe that was why he didn't work a regular ward. It seems he was put where staff numbers were reduced on any given day. I worry that those poor tied-up ladies dreaded seeing him at 7:00am.

The other category of staff were the homely, kind, thoughtful and compassionate individuals who turned up to do their best each and every day; they were the cheerful ones, the ones that sang whilst going about their work, the ones who hugged the ladies and held their hands, and the ones that appeared to love the ladies as if they were their own families.

I am not talking about the qualified staff here either, as these were often the auxiliary nurses, not formally qualified, but with so much experience working in these challenging environments. I discovered in time that many of these kind folks were often from the same families, generations of families having worked in the hospital for years in one role or another. However, despite their kindness, they still tied legs to chairs and bathed three different ladies in the bathrooms with no screens and one bar of soap and a flannel between them. "You finished with the soap? Chuck it over then." It was so cold in the bathing area, Brrrrrr, we in our centrally heated homes cannot imagine it now! Those poor ladies were heaved out of the warm water to be dried with the thinnest, smallest towels you can imagine, and they would go to the next kind person who would dress them from their allocated 'bundle'.

The bundles were made up by the night staff (or were supposed to have been!), and they were put together in the laundry room, and each lady had a bundle for the next day. I did bundles many times: a dress made of crimplene, a cardigan, a pair of cotton knickers, a pair of stockings and a vest. I often wondered if any of the ladies actually wore the same outfit more than once! Whether the lady was tall or short, large or slim, more or less, they got what they were given.

Sometimes if someone looked nice in, say, pink, then we would try to give her pink, but the dresses could possibly trip you up if too long and big or show your bum if too small to wrap around you properly. If a garment was particularly washed out or needed mending, it would be put in a bag for the sewing room, after which it would be put back into circulation once mended. I used to quite like doing the bundles, especially if I was on my own because I could hide away in that warm room and do my best to get clothes together which I thought would fit and suit each lady. That didn't happen very often though, as it was thought of as skiving if you took too long doing it. I learned a great deal on that ward, especially about how routines ruled the days. I learned too that to hope these people would have the chance of a slightly different and more fulfilling life before they die, then I would have to be very brave, very strong and also realistic about the possibility of introducing change. Also, I would also need to be very mindful of what these ladies actually wanted and were able to manage.

You see, the condition of 'institutionalisation' was cruel, damaging, and demoralising but also safe and unchallenging for some who had settled into a daily routine for many years, knowing what to expect and when. Rocking the boat or introducing change or even the opportunity for having choice could be extremely scary for them. Politicians and activists were working outside the asylum to instigate change, but when you are actually working there, wrapped up in firm and long-established daily routines, well, that was a different story. On reflection, we were aware that change was needed and didn't agree with many of the practices and treatments in those days, but had to be patient and comply to a degree. In order to implement change from within, which can often be more effective than protesting from outside, we had to be seen to 'play the game' to earn position, power and respect in order to be able to institute change. This had to be worth it for the sake of the then patients and for the care of others in the future.

'THE GERIATRIC WARD'

Yes, believe it or not, this was a term used for my next ward experience and nowadays would be considered a somewhat derogatory term meaning 'decrepit' or 'outdated'. Some years later we adopted a more acceptable term for this type of ward, which was 'Care of the Elderly'.

Reuniting with my fellow students in school felt like meeting again with long-lost friends who all had just experienced something very similar. We shared our experiences, socialised together and felt we all had gained quite an insight into what were called in those days 'mental illnesses'. I felt that my own life had taken on a more positive vibe. My children were quite settled in school and nursery, and I am sure that they gained some benefit from having a more fulfilled mother. My husband was still working at a local garage, so he too was in an employment routine. He did sometimes forget to pick his own child up from school if I was on a late shift, and I would get a frantic call from a teacher asking who should be picking up a very distressed little boy. I knew deep down in my heart that my other half was still quite unreliable, often wrapped up in his own things, so I recruited my parents whenever possible to help out with childcare. I was determined to try and see this training through to the end and know I couldn't have done it without my long-suffering parents. Three cheers for grandparents.

Back in school we started to learn more about the physical and practical care of a patient, encompassing care of the elderly and dying. This involved everything from basic feeding, washing and dressing a patient to performing physical tests, aseptic techniques, care of diabetes, coronary care, epilepsy, and terminal care. We even learned how to evacuate patients who were ill or unable to walk from a multistorey building in the case of fire. This involved a great deal of fun by strapping each other to mattresses and bumping each other down the stairs at high speed. This was not exactly how it should be done, but the fireman teaching us lost control at one point, as we had reverted to being children in a playground and were tearing upstairs and downstairs, saying, "Again, it's my turn next; this is so much fun." The reality of trying to evacuate elderly, sick or confused patients down flights of stairs, in the case of fire, would be a very different story, but we got the gist of what to do.

Anatomy and physiology were drummed into our brains, so we used many mnemonics to remember names of muscle groups or cranial nerves, and some inventive students created rude poems or songs to remember things. Those methods worked very well. We were being prepared to deal with all manner of physical illnesses, as patients who have mental health problems, like the general public, often have physical illnesses too, especially the elderly.

Our next two ward experiences were to be spent on an elderly ward and then a long stay ward. Most of the latter, at that time, were undergoing massive changes to introduce rehabilitation programmes as a solution to the massive problem of institutionalisation, which is easier said than done, as anyone who spends longer than only a week in hospital finds themself experiencing symptoms of institutionalisation very quickly. So 30 years in the institution takes some undoing, which I will discuss later on, but first I was heading to a 'geriatric ward', as it would be called in those days.

So once again with my stiff uniform back on, I arrived on my allocated ward to see 'a sea' of white-haired old ladies, mainly in chairs, all looking exactly the same. Panic set in because I immediately thought, "How will I tell one from the other?" Then I was distracted by the sharp ammonia smell of stale urine, mixed with the smell of old mashed potato and slightly masked by a smell of strong disinfection. It really turned my stomach at first, but I was then greeted by the sister on the ward and summoned to the office to be introduced to the ward. The sister was friendly and helpful enough but seemed distracted by the need to get out on the ward and help, as there was so much to do. The general atmosphere was noisy, with patients crying out, staff shouting to each other and wheelchairs being pushed at speed to and from toilets or bathrooms. I was escorted to one of the large dormitories and introduced to a second-year nursing student who would be working with me and 'showing me the ropes'. We had forty beds to make and three dressings to perform on three ladies who appeared to be quite poorly and were permanently in bed.

The young nurse was friendly with a good sense of humour, and we got to know each other well whilst making all those beds, chatting about our lives and sharing information. She proceeded to turn the radio up, dance, sing and wear one of the patient's liberty bodices supporting four dangling suspenders over her uniform whilst working. I later learned that after spending day after day doing the same activities, larking about was a good distraction to help get through the day. The dressing trolley was prepared, and I was initiated into the aseptic technique of performing a dressing, which involved me being the dirty nurse, opening the packages and touching the outside of things, whilst my colleague, wearing gloves and using tweezers, only touched the sterile areas which were on the inside of the dressing pack. The poor patient in the bed was an emaciated elderly lady with contracted limbs and a huge bed sore on her hip, which was deep and smelly. We worked together cleaning the wound and packing it with dressings. It was horrible, as it was obvious that the lady was in dreadful pain as we touched her and tried to make her more comfortable. It was explained to me that she was already prescribed morphine and was probably not going to get better. She didn't respond to our talking to her and just stared hauntingly at us. The other two elderly ladies in the dormitory were in a similar predicament. I felt really upset and worried about them when I went home, wishing I could have comforted them more somehow.

I asked what had caused such terrible wounds, and my fellow colleague explained that these were bed or pressure sores caused by lying or sitting in bed for too long in the same position. This could cause the normal blood flow to restrict, and when a patient is emaciated, unable to move themselves and not healthy or well nourished, the skin can break down under pressure. This was seen as the product of bad nursing because a patient in this predicament should be regularly turned or moved to relieve pressure on certain areas of the body. Bony areas like heels, elbows, hips and shoulders are very susceptible to sores. My thoughts were, "Had these three ladies been left and ignored for too long in bed without movement?" And I think that the answer, sadly, was probably yes. With so many needy patients, few staff and so much to do, the quiet ones in bed, unable to move, were forgotten or left until there was time to deal with them. Fortunately we students were around to tend to these patients while the regular staff got on with all the other tasks, but for these three ladies it was a bit too late, as their recovery was unlikely.

As the weeks went on I spent most of my days in the same dormitory with the young student nurse doing the same tasks every day in addition to some feeding of helpless patients and helping with bathing. I did get to know patients' names and recognise the large differences between them. I discovered their different personalities and also learned some very rude swear words, which I had never heard before, let alone used myself, coming out of the mouths of 'sweet' little old ladies. In all honesty, if I were living out the last of my days in this place, I would probably let rip and swear a great deal. Life was just routine, and there was not much time for pleasure. I began to get used to unpleasant smells and didn't really notice them. We became very close to the three very ill ladies in our dormitory whom we cared for every day and held their hands, talking and even singing to them on occasions. When one of them sadly died, I stayed with her and held her hand to the end, but will never get over the fact many of them had no outside friends or relatives to come and comfort them. Mental illness carried such a stigma that many families forgot about their suffering relatives, as they couldn't face up to, or perhaps understand, how valuable a visit from a friend or relative can be to someone in hospital. We all benefit from knowing someone cares about us, don't we?

In general the staff were kind and friendly, but my student friend and I soon realised that we were often given tasks out of the way from the rest of the activities on the ward, to keep us busy because some staff felt quite threatened by us 'students' coming in from school with all these 'new ideas' and views, which were often about putting the patient first and not the routine. One staff nurse who I had great respect for was a very posh middle-aged woman who called everyone 'darling' and was so kind to all the patients even when they swore at her or lashed out. She was always immaculate, cheerful and really helpful and supportive to us students. On the other hand, one of the State Enrolled Nurses, who was not far from her retirement, was horrible to the patients, shouting at them, rushing them and being quite rough, which really upset me, and I was on the point of reporting her to someone, but I didn't know how or to whom. I was terrified of her. She was a bully. She talked in the staff room quite openly to an audience of us nurses about her marriage and referred to her husband as 'it'. They were living separate lives, and she was hoping he would die so she could have the house to herself.

She was one of the old staff who never did any formal training but had been awarded the State Enrolled Nurse status for working many years as an auxiliary nurse. This had been a regular practice in the past because there was a massive shortage of trained nurses to take charge. They were known as 'made up SENs'. I think many had a large chip on their shoulder because they felt worried or threatened that the new trained SENs may see gaps in their knowledge. This particular nurse made it very clear that she hated us students and didn't want to hear one word out of our mouths! Some time later I was not sorry to hear she had been suspended from duty and later asked to leave. I also realised that she had her own mental health issues, as we all have to different degrees, but taking your frustrations out on poor frail elderly patients was just not on. I will talk later on about some of the 'madness', hilarity and unusual characters amongst the staff. Many fitted in well to the environment of the large psychiatric hospital, and their oddities were unnoticed there, as they would have probably been in the outside world of work.

The whole experience on this ward was very enlightening and very different from my last ward. I learned so much more from it. Despite the very hard physical work, it was very rewarding too. The reward was helping people to be more comfortable or making them smile, which is a small but very huge thing under those circumstances. The routine ruled, making the ward run by the clock but not necessarily for the comfort of the patient. There were books to record weekly bathing, opening of bowels, spending patient's money on their behalf, etc. These were all controlled by the nurse in charge for that shift, who carried a large bunch of keys, and everything was locked, so in order to get a new pair of stockings or tights for someone, you had to ask the nurse in charge.

I became aware over the weeks that these wards were still very much run as the old institution was for many years by older, more mature staff, but change was coming. We students were being encouraged in school to question everything. Why do we do things this way, or what are the benefits to the patient? One buzzword of the time was 'institutionalisation', which was seen as a very destructive condition itself caused by, as I mentioned previously, spending long periods of time locked in an institution, mainly run by strict rules with little space for choice or individuality, which brings me on to the long stay wards and 'rehabilitation', another buzzword of those times.

So I continued to work on various wards, usually eight weeks on each, sometimes with four-week spells back in the school of nursing to learn and gain more knowledge, which hopefully helped me to become a better and more experienced nurse. One of the main lessons that always stuck with me was to question everything. Things had been done in the institution the same way for many years, and we were living in a time of change from the 60s to the 70s and onwards, not only in society but also in medical and psychological research. As a result, new recruits to the professions working in mental health were quite a revolutionary lot, especially in nursing.

It was Health Minister Enoch Powell who argued that mental hospitals were effectively prisons and they prevented a return to normal life outside the walls. The introduction of improved psychotropic drugs in the late 1960s meant that gradually there may be a better chance to treat people away from the institutions. And during the 1970s large-scale psychiatric hospitals were being discredited, and a societal change in attitudes was supported by charities and civil rights movements. However, as suggested, it was the staff within those institutions who took the lead from within to instigate change. It was a difficult role, met with a mixture of excited, positive attitudes to the changes with plenty of scepticism and fear.

We revolutionary nurses were very much in the thick of it, and we had to learn very quickly how to introduce new ideas and ways of treatment, taking into account patient needs, not the needs of the institution. As previously mentioned, there was a difference between the admissions ward and the older persons' wards. I will continue to reflect upon this, as it clearly demonstrated how we new, visionary nurses had to carefully pick our times and our people to continue striving for a different world for the people behind those walls, as not all were on board, especially those in charge.

In 1983 the introduction of legislation which gave the mentally ill more rights, allowing them to appeal against committal, arrived to support our quest in the form of the *1983 Mental Health Act*{2}. But we were working and trying to instigate change in much earlier days… and damn it, we had just got to grips with the *1959 Mental Health Act*{1}. So it was necessary for all staff to learn the new legislation and what changes had been made. Also the rights of patients and the process of appealing against a decision had been reviewed in favour of the individual being detained.

So in the next chapter Debbi relates her experiences whilst working on her first admission ward in the hospital, which was for her like entering a completely different world.

ENTERING A DIFFERENT WORLD

The admission ward was at the front of the hospital; it had been upgraded and was actually quite modern for its day. There was a different vibe there; it was busy, efficient and more professional somehow.

I was greeted by a ward sister who told me that I was there to learn and would not be expected to take part in the more mundane tasks on the ward, such as bed making. Haha! Kidding, aren't you!

I worked so hard on that ward, but there we go again; I was being swept up into the breeze of change that was permanently there like electricity somehow. Evidently Angela was feeling the same and seeing a new way to do things emerging, kicking against the old institutional ways of doing things. When we first met, that's when I knew; it was almost like an unspoken mission! To understand what was going on in our world of work and how we were going to shape it, not just then but in the future too.

One of my first recollections of that placement was of an elderly lady, very small, grey-haired and wearing a floral apron which was down to her shins. She was brought by an ambulance to the ward. She was terrified, a tragic and pathetic sight to see. She was twisting her hands around each other, she was very pale, her eyes were like saucers in her little face, and she was weeping.

I had been told that her husband had passed away approximately six months previously, and since then she had become a recluse; her self-care was poor and her neighbours had been worried about her not being seen for some time. The police had broken in and found her home in a poor state. She had not been eating or drinking very much; she was very thin, and there was a dead cat in the kitchen, which was attracting a lot of flies. The admissions room on the ward was not unpleasant; it was bright, the examination bed had a clean sheet on it, and there was a desk and two chairs on the opposite wall. A small window offered a little fresh air, which was needed as the poor lady smelled badly. She also had head lice, and her skin was very dry and gradually shedding from her bare reddish-blue legs underneath the crimplene skirt that she was wearing, underneath the apron. We were tasked with helping her to undress and to go to the bathroom to have a bath and to be given some clean nightwear. This was what patients wore when newly admitted. The lady was very frightened and held on to her clothes for dear life, so it took us a long time to gently persuade her to remove them; they were in rags, really, and badly soiled. However, this was when we had a huge shock! We noticed that the seams on virtually every item were misshapen and 'fat'; they had been resewn too. All around the floral apron, her cardigan and the hem of her tatty old skirt, her old shoes, which were once fur-lined, I think, were very sloppy on her feet, actually far too big for her. They were men's boots, it turned out, and the front of them were tightly stuffed with rolled-up money! Her hems and seams, so carefully sewn, were also full of rolled-up notes!

No wonder she did not want to let go of her clothes! Needless to say, we were very shocked, and when we began to slowly unpick the stitching with the lady present at all times, we began to develop quite a pile of notes on the desk. It was at this point we went to get the charge nurse, who called for a security man from the front gate to guard it whilst suited men from goodness knows where appeared to take charge.

If I remember correctly, the lady had thousands of pounds sewn into her garments, bless her. As a mere student, I was never made aware of what happened to that lady in terms of the rest of her life. She was still on the ward when I left, but she had improved; she was very quiet and much less frightened, and I am pleased to tell you she had a regular visitor too. I think it was a niece who always stayed a while, and the lady seemed pleased to see her.

Yes, this is actually a good example of the changes that were coming into the mental health services in the UK at the time. If you compare the experience of the admission ward to the experience of my first ward, commonly known as a 'back ward' (not sure why, but forgotten; I think possibly 'not as important and hidden in the background' fits), this felt more hopeful; yes, patients had visitors and also a bedside locker! I believe these were the first tentative steps towards change, and if you read my friend's chapter about her experience, even uniforms were being ditched!

I recall a day which I will never forget on that ward. It was a day which I think sums up the relationships we made with colleagues and the sense of devilment which has never left me. I cannot recall whether it was due to striking (there was a lot of unrest and shortages and subsequent strikes during this time) or petrol shortage, but the ward clerk on this ward was due to see her boyfriend, and she had no fuel in her car, a very distressing situation for her! The nurses, however, were allowed to get fuel, so, the kind person that I am, I said she could borrow my uniform at lunchtime and go to the garage. So we went into a dormitory, and I stripped off. I am five foot two inches, and she was about five foot ten inches; we did not think of this when we hatched our plan! However, mini skirts were quite fashionable! The plan was, I would hide in the dormitory (sleeping area) while she did the quick ten-minute trip to get fuel. I was wearing my underwear and my cape, thinking about putting on her extra-long trousers when I heard a male patient approaching. He was shouting "Fuck off" repeatedly; this was due to Tourette's syndrome. I knew he would be upset if he saw me in the dormitory at lunchtime (routines were important, remember!). So I rolled underneath the bed quickly, but Bobby saw me, and sadly I left the long trousers on the top of the bed. Next thing I heard above the man shouting his swear word was another nurse calling him, "Bobby, come on, you know you should not be here. Matron is coming, so please come back to the day room." OH NO! I forgot Matron was due to come to the ward to do her inspection! Bobby was getting more and more worked up; he was screaming and shouting, so I took my chance and got out of a window (the windows were locked but opened to air the dorms after cleaning). Poor Bobby! He was so upset, but Matron and a colleague arrived and managed to remove him. The matron voiced her displeasure and told my colleague to "get these windows locked NOW". There was me now outside, wearing very little, and panicking because I should be on the ward for inspection! I could see the car park from behind the bush I was hiding behind, and I saw the ward clerk approaching and parking up. I shouted at her as loud as I could dare, and she thankfully wandered calmly to my bush. We both ran to the safety of her car and swapped clothes. Except, of course, for her trousers! We agreed that I would tell the sister that she was feeling unwell and was sitting in her car hoping the nausea would pass. I just had to somehow get her trousers out to her before someone saw her! I am smiling to myself as I write this; it sounds like something from a Carry On film! (if you are old enough to know what they were, if not, google it!) I managed to get one of the auxiliary nurses to go and get the trousers and take them out undetected. Hilarious! Later during the evening when all was quiet, I explained to Bobby what had gone on; he just gave me a small smile and walked away. Not sure he believed me, to be honest!

I recall doing an assessment of a new admission on this ward, which highlights how things could go wrong and the need to have the courage to speak up when, as a student nurse, you do as the doctor says. A lady was struggling with anxiety and had been sent for assessment by her GP. She had her daughter with her, and the only available room was small; I had to stand up behind the doctor, who sat at the desk taking his notes. The doctor was Asian, and he had quite a strong accent. Very early in the assessment, the lady said, "It is raining cats and dogs out there." I noticed he had written that 'she sees cats and dogs coming from the sky.' Inevitably the assessment was going in the wrong direction. The doctor was considering the possibility of psychosis, and the questioning was upsetting the lady; her daughter became upset, saying, "My mum is not mad; we need to get out of here."

I quietly pointed out to the doctor that the statement made about cats and dogs was actually a metaphor, and he had misunderstood. Unfortunately, he did not respond very positively, and the assessment was abandoned when the daughter took her mum home. I never did get the opportunity to sit with the doctor and explain properly, but it worried me that if the daughter had not intervened, that lady's life may have been very different going forward.

Even today, you can still see the division between 'old psychiatry' and 'new psychiatry', but the gap is thankfully getting smaller, as patients who experienced old psychiatry (which was mainly underpinned by an attitude of when you go into the asylum, you will never get out) are largely dying out, and patients who have benefitted from much improved science and treatment options with the belief that recovery is possible are now experiencing mental health services in a very different way. Today, hope is a key foundation, whereas in the '70s it did not really exist for individuals who had been incarcerated for sometimes 30-40 years.

'THE LOCKED WARD'

Back to life as a student nurse in the 1970s/'80s. My next placement was on a male locked ward. Angela recalls working for a short time before her training, on the same ward, but at that time it was a female ward, and when we chatted about our work (as we frequently did), it seemed very little had changed.

It was here I became familiar with lots of difficult issues, which also gave me a learning opportunity which was to stand me in good stead for the rest of my career. The gentlemen on this ward were very seriously and chronically unwell. I vividly remember the layout and smells of this smaller, dark, dismal and noisy ward. My first thoughts were that it felt very unpredictable. Staff were confident but also wary and on high alert all the time. Assessing risk was high on the agenda, and it soon became apparent that the staff knew their patients well, and they also cared about them. They cared about how they were dressed, how they were fed, and most of all, they cared about maintaining a safe environment (at least as safe as it could be made).

There were three policy 20 rooms on this ward, horrible cells with mattresses on the floor. The walls were stained with what I was told was faeces, which was scrubbed and washed regularly. There was more than one man who frequently smeared the walls in these rooms with his own faeces when he was locked in there for his own safety and the safety of others. Jim, as I shall call one of the men, would become very distressed by his voices, pacing around screaming at them to "Fuck off and leave me alone!" He would claw at his ears and head, making himself bleed. A consequence of this would be a high dose of an injectable antipsychotic called Haloperidol; it would calm his voices, but the side effects were awful for him. He suffered from some oculogyric crises, which meant the muscles around his eyes would involuntarily pull his eyes up into his head as if he was straining to look upwards; it must have been so painful for him and quite shocking to witness.

I remember he would try to walk with very stiff limbs, arms outstretched to stop himself walking into walls; he was agitated and frightened. The poor man would be calling out, "Need an injection, nurse, need an injection."

Other patients on the ward did not like this; the atmosphere became quite hostile, some shouting at him to "Shut the fuck up" and others shouting at staff to "Do something with him! Lock him up."

The drill was: a qualified member of staff would prepare the injection of Kemadrin, a drug which helped counteract the severe side effects sometimes suffered from taking major tranquilliser medication. Then two other staff members would approach him with a bed sheet stretched out between them and literally trap him in the sheet and quickly wrap his arms in it and wrestle him to the floor. Two other staff would then restrain him with their weight on his shoulders, hips and ankles whilst the qualified staff would inject him. The whole process was swift and well-practised. When it was safe to do so, he would be helped, still in the sheet, to his feet, and he was put in the room with the mattress, and the door was securely locked. A staff member was then outside the door for however long it took for him to calm down and eventually go to sleep. I remember doing this and having to record every five minutes how he was behaving and whether he was 'safe'. I remember the section of his case file where these notes were filed was thick and scruffy; the paper was marked with the fingerprints of the staff who had sat on a chair outside that room so often. He had been in that room many times, poor chap.

The long-term staff on the ward (I was to become one of them at a later date) always took care of him after one of these episodes. He was gently bathed in warm soapy bubbles to ease his sore limbs and wash off the faeces; he was then put to sleep on one of the mattresses in a policy room (if they were not in use) so that he could sleep without being disturbed by other patients. He was given a pillow and warm blankets.

People used to say to me, "How do you do it?", "Don't you get scared?" The answer is no… I felt threatened very few times in all my career, but these times have been due to illness, not badness.

The layout of this ward did not really lend itself to staff safety! I have absolutely no doubt that today it would shut down. There were dormitories upstairs, and the stairs were down at the bottom of a dark narrow corridor. Generally patients were not allowed upstairs during the day, but one day someone had made a mistake and the door was left unlocked. Everything was locked on this ward. On this day I went up to the linen cupboard. Why did I not think it was odd that the door was unlocked? No idea! But off I went, in a rush as usual, no doubt! Suddenly I was confronted by a man who was extremely paranoid. He believed that everyone was against him and that people disliked him, thinking that he looked like a monkey. I recall he actually looked a bit like the convicted murderer Peter Sutcliffe! And he had a razor blade in his hand, and he was standing about a foot away from me… … "Did you just say I looked like a monkey?" Yes, I was frightened at the time. I knew nobody would hear me if I screamed, I knew I should not have gone up there on my own without checking that it was safe, and I knew I was in big trouble. I thought that I could maybe back into one of the bathroom cubicles and use my weight against the door if I could reach one of the baths with my short legs! No chance! He kept asking if I thought he looked like a monkey, and of course I kept denying it! I tried using his name a lot, and I think I kept my voice outwardly calm - de-escalation, they call it today! Then in a wonky/distorted non-glass mirror on the wall above one of the sinks, I saw my saviour! I saw a man who had arrived in the UK some months before and became very unwell, and he was being treated for a psychotic illness. He very calmly said in a broad African accent, "You got trouble, blondie?"

This gave me the opportunity to duck, and run like hell! Back down the stairs shouting for colleagues to help. Thinking back, there were two staff halfway there, probably wondering where I had disappeared to! I knew my African saviour would be safe; he was a huge man! As broad as he was tall, and little 'Peter Sutcliffe' did not stand a chance, blade or no blade!

Seriously, I learned many lessons that day which I have taken with me throughout my long career. Always listen; listen to your heart; respect people who have more experience than you; listen to them. Why are they saying these things? Work it out. What are your options? Why? Where? Who? Listen and ask all the time, work it out… But if your heart says yes, then go ahead if it is for the good of the person you are caring for. POSITIVE RISKS! Oh my God, have I taken so many of those positive risks in my career!

Hahaha, I am so proud of that. I really have stuck my neck out for the individuals I worked with, and I carried on doing that as long as I kept working. Bugger the establishment and rules; if it is right, just do it … sod it!

There were many practices to be questioned on this ward, mostly depending on who was in charge. I was doing a medication round one day with 'a qualified' and he asked me if I had a cough. No… "Yes, you have," he replied, and he showed me how when I 'coughed', I would pour more Largactil into the tumbler which held the brown, thick liquid. (Largactil, or chlorpromazine, is an antipsychotic medication which actually means 'large acting'; it acts on all parts of the brain, and subsequently the side effects were horrible: excess salivation, drooling, rigid limbs, restlessness, literally not being able to keep still, drowsiness and the previously mentioned oculogyric crisis). These were the visible effects, but the heart, liver and kidneys also suffered.

Every man on this ward was given large doses of this drug; the bottle on the trolley was huge, and when new, I could barely lift it with one hand to measure, though measuring was far from accurate! The small plastic measuring cups which held 20 ml were useless, and as I said, it was given in plastic tumblers, and the dose literally was guesswork. Unbelievable, but the men queued up for it three / four times a day.

Meal times also meant a queue at the trolley. One chap who had been on the locked ward for 25 years or more had a ritual… He would come to the trolley to get two sausages for breakfast; he then scampered across the room, moved a chair and lifted the corner of the carpet. The sausages were put there, and he returned to the trolley to get toast and porridge, all the time watching the corner of the room, keeping guard of his precious sausages. He would take his toast and porridge, sit on the chair and eat his food, tipping the bowl to drink the porridge.

He would then toss (not throw) the bowl, hoping someone would pick it up (staff always did, as it was a potential weapon); he would then sit on the chair until he wanted to retrieve the sausages and eat them. Do not even begin to think of the years of sausage fat, grime, dust and cockroach poo that was under that carpet!

Sadly sometimes someone, sometimes even staff, would tease him and pretend to try to get his sausages. This was very cruel. I am sure there have been times, years before, that he would not have had food to eat at all, and he developed this ritual to survive in his mind. If he was challenged, he became very, very angry. He was a small but strong, wiry man, and there was no controlling him without the sheet and medication restraint. I witnessed on two occasions, when someone decided to have some 'sport', his friend on the ward, who was the biggest man I had ever seen, with hands like dinner plates and standing about three feet taller, picked up the cruel individual and threw him at the wall. He then walked away. There was no help for the teaser and no punishment for the sausage-hiding man. I would call this in-house management, and it was fair in my view. Served him right.

I was on that ward for approximately two years later on, and I think to witness this twice suggests nobody dared tease that guy very often!

Exercise and fresh air on this ward was in an enclosed area off the ward, but sometimes we would take a man for a walk in the grounds on a ratio of 2:1 minimum. I used to enjoy this, as the men really seemed to also. Sometimes they would have to wear pyjamas to do this in case they absconded and it would be obvious they were from the hospital. Nobody attempted to do this when I was with them.

We once filled bin bags with snow when we had deep snow and went 'plackybaggin'! Cheap improvised sledges. Hilarious, great fun. I remember some of the smiles of those men! With their brown-stained teeth or toothless mouths and yellowing skin. They did not have the chance to laugh very often, but when they did, it was so good to see. But as they were only in pyjamas and an old overcoat, we couldn't stay long!

I recall thinking many times how strange it must be to never have physical contact with another human, unless being restrained. I am a very huggy person. I like to give hugs and receive them, but these men (and all the women I came in contact with on those 'back-wards') had probably not been touched for years. How very, very sad. I make a point to always shake hands with patients; some female patients I will put an arm around a shoulder or even hug, but always, at a minimum, I will shake hands. I don't worry if those hands are dirty, stained with nicotine and with very long fingernails; you cannot catch schizophrenia from physical contact!

I believe it shows respect, and although sometimes there is an element of surprise, my hand has never been refused.

The locked ward taught me so much about mental illness, mental health law, professionalism and respect. I will never forget it, and I took the strength to believe in change being possible with me to work every day. Never give up believing that one can try to make things better. Ever.

It was on this ward that I was due to spend my first Christmas away from home; I was sad that day. However, at 8.30 the charge nurse asked if I had ten pence. I answered yes, and he said, "Go and phone your father and tell him to come and get you; come back for tea time tomorrow." I could not believe it! I phoned Dad, who willingly came for me. It took him away from the family for about four hours in all, but it was worth it! I shall never forget this; it was such a kind and thoughtful gesture. I recall staff and some of the men waving and shouting "Happy Christmas" as I left the ward.

REHABILITATION?

So Debbi certainly was starting to taste different aspects of the types of care given on varied wards in the hospital and gaining many thoughts or feelings around this. Like me, her head was full of questions, and she felt touched by what she had seen and heard. I then having experienced the admission ward with patients in acute, recent phases of their 'mental illnesses' as they were called in those days, and then experiencing a 'geriatric ward' with patients who had spent most of their lives in the psychiatric hospital, having just become elderly or some having developed 'mental illness' in later life, was next introduced to a totally different experience on 'The Rehabilitation Ward'.

Rehabilitation of long stay, institutionalised patients in large mental hospitals was a new and exciting venture with a view to discharging many patients back into the community to lead a normal life. All sounds fairly straightforward, but as mentioned previously, many patients had been in hospital for many years in a very structured environment with little choice and no voice or opinion, and everything was provided by the institution and its staff. So often the reasons they had found themselves in the hospital initially had long gone, some having recovered from a mental health problem or some being there wrongly because they didn't fit in with society's or their family's expectations. Many of these individuals were now suffering from another condition to varying degrees called Institutionalisation. Symptoms of this condition could include strange repetitive mannerisms, inability to make decisions, lack of knowledge of the modern world, loss of speech and loss of confidence. Also, long-term use of tranquilising medication had left many with serious side effects.

The fact that in the aim of caring for individuals or protecting them from a dreadful life in their community or the workhouse, to take you back to the history of the hospital, we had unknowingly created major problems for many people. So Rehabilitation to combat Institutionalisation entailed trying to teach people a different way of living, where they could have their own named clothes, have money, go shopping, learn to cook, learn to socialise, and learn to use a launderette or modern appliance. The list is endless of all the things we take for granted in a modern life.

I arrived at the ward, which was called a 'house' to move away from the word 'hospital'. I was introduced to the sister in charge and another student nurse who was in her final year of training. We wore mufti, or our own clothes, for work. We were encouraged to allow the 'residents', not 'patients', to get on with things as much as possible on their own. There was a weekly timetable of activities which we supervised. Some of the residents went out to occupational or industrial therapy during the week, so we hung around in a practically empty building some of the time.

We were charged with teaching the patients all about decimal currency, some cooking, shopping trips, going out for meals, going to the cinema or the pub, using money and helping with personal care or care of each person's individual room. This is all well and good in theory, but probably most individuals need teaching how to do all these daily living skills well, especially some nurses and doctors! We were being trained as nurses, not teachers, so our imparting of knowledge to these residents was based totally on our own experiences of life. Thankfully, having been thrown into married life very young and having to bring up a family, I was familiar with the practical side of coping and daily living. Alternatively, that would not necessarily be the case for many of the other young student nurses who, as young people away from home for the first time, didn't always look after themselves very well, but they certainly would have had more ideas than those poor institutionalised patients.

Eventually, if all went well, some individuals were discharged to group homes or hostels or homes for the elderly in the community. Not many went back to their own family or lived independently. Sadly their families had long gone or stopped all contact with them, and they were being discharged into a community who didn't want them with their strange mannerisms or history of 'mental problems' due to lack of knowledge or understanding. Prejudice was rife at that time, and although some of the public were kind and thought it was good to allow people back into the community after all these years in hospital, they didn't particularly want a group home next door to them.

Another problem was that some long-term patients didn't want their life to change. The hospital had been their home for most of their adult life. They felt safe and knew what to expect every day, as life was predictable. There was sometimes a resistance to trying to learn new things, and during my time working there, I saw some have a complete relapse due to the stress of being pushed too much towards discharge. Others even attempted suicide, so it was a very serious and sensitive business.

Another interesting fact was that all the time I was there for my eight-week placement, I only saw the sister come out of her office about three times. She never trained us or taught us anything and had many visitors who went into her office for hours, and the door was shut. I learned much later on in my career that the whiskey bottle came out a great deal! So my student colleague and I just got on with it in our own inexperienced way. We took the residents out and about in small groups and encouraged them to make choices, spend money and have fun. Some embraced it, but others just sat there and waited to be told what to do.

We encouraged them to use our Christian names, but they would shout in a cafe, "Nurse, can I smoke in here?" or "Nurse, can we go back to the ward?" They just weren't ready, sadly. We tried our best but felt we were wasting our time sometimes and enjoyed the times when we had nothing to do, so we could chat and amuse ourselves. Nobody really cared what we were up to!

Despite all this, some residents did move out into group homes in groups of four and had the support of community nurses and social workers. They worked fairly well but often had the usual problems of multi-occupancy when compromise was necessary and mental health workers were called in to help keep the peace. Those who went to live in hostels or homes for the elderly settled quite well, probably because they went into another less controlling institution where they felt safe and cared for. Also the 'mental illness' label was thankfully removed.

The hospital had other Rehabilitation schemes happening too at the same time, one being a Token Economy Ward where patients were rewarded for various simple achievements. Psychologists were involved in selecting patients for this. Token Economy was based on research which showed that people can repeatedly perform well when rewarded. On the lines of Pavlov's dog research? Or maybe sadly, bribery sometimes works to get what you want and is used to help solve crimes when prisoners are offered better conditions in exchange for information. Human behaviour does respond to fairly basic temptations. I don't know how successful the scheme was with long stay psychiatric patients, but the unit was later closed, having been an experiment which wasn't very effective. As said previously, it was a time of change, and there was much effort to help undo many of the old institutional ways of treating mental health problems, with a view to reducing the vast number of patients in the hospital and finding ways of discharging as many as possible back into the community.

Finally, another approach was tried on two wards down at The Annex. With Rehabilitation in mind, patients were selected with a view to discharge at a later date. The wards were run as a therapeutic community, where inmates could manage their own lives as much as possible. They were encouraged to make choices about daily activities, manage their own medication if able, answer the ward telephone and, with the staff's guidance or help, make decisions. They had group meetings and were encouraged to speak their mind. There was a high ratio of staff, and they were seen by other ward staff to be having an easy life, leaving everything up to the patients, even ordering laundry, meals, etc.

Many were discharged to group homes, and the staff from the ward went out to visit them to give support and provide continuity of care.

Interestingly, that unit was also closed. New management arrived and was unable to cope with all the rules being scrapped, i.e., the nurses weren't in control, so all sorts of safety issues were raised. The laundry, kitchens and pharmacy didn't like dealing with patients when they phoned the ward. They complained that nurses should answer the phone. So the institution felt challenged and fought back. All that really mattered is that many patients were discharged and were living in the community, hopefully living happier lives. Also there would no longer be hundreds of 'long stay' patients locked in wards for the rest of their lives in large institutions. The population numbers at the hospital were slowly reducing due to discharge from the rehabilitation programme, also just old age leading to death and the new attitudes or treatments for new admissions who were discharged back home mainly at the earliest opportunity.

Interestingly, looking around today at our 'crisis in mental health' affected by things like a diagnosis of autism or ADHD, violence, homelessness, poverty, drug abuse, knife crime, screen addiction and many other modern-day life issues, it begs the question, will we need large institutions in the future to house and 'look after' all these struggling individuals and victims of their mental health crises? In view of the fact that many don't feel there is any help for them out there and the current services are overstretched, I really hope not and don't really believe that large hospitals are the answer.

Or are these modern-day life and social issues a product of the way we live in our modern society, and when experiencing any of these life problems, people's reactions to them are to be expected as they are traumatic? So does society need to recognise this and change some of its behaviour? Maybe a good place to start is with what we teach and introduce our children to in life at a very young age. They are introduced to screens whilst still in their prams. They had Covid to deal with. Evidently many are struggling with basic life skills. What is acceptable behaviour, and what are the basic needs and rights of every human being? What are the simple things that make us happy? What is wrong with showing kindness and helping others? How do we deal with our feelings? Many questions with some simple answers, but very important to address if we want to live in a mentally healthy society.

FURTHER MEMORIES

There were some continuations of the same sorts of experiences already mentioned, but other things that still spring to mind are the events that stay in my memory for various reasons. As previously mentioned, due to changes in ideas regarding training and views on part-time working, I, Angela, must have done the longer spell of training than most, for four and a half years, to become a Registered Mental Nurse, but it gave me the opportunity to have a great deal of varied experience, during which time I got to know many nurses and patients at the hospital and made very good lifelong friends, such as Debbi, who by then had become a close friend, and we regularly shared our thoughts and feelings about work when we were together. We never actually worked on the same ward, but as you can tell by relating memories, we had a great deal in common, experiencing many similar things.

For example, I worked on another elderly female ward down at The Annex, which was a smaller set of buildings similar to the main hospital, situated about a mile down the road. Debbi has already recounted her experiences on her first ward there. I was once told in jest by a male nurse that if you were banished to the annex, either as a patient or staff member, you were changed forever or sometimes never seen again! Not understanding whether this was a joke or why he said this was enough to make a rather green second-year student nurse a bit nervous about her first 'annex' experience.

A male nurse whom I knew had left the hospital to emigrate to Australia for a few years and was asked by a colleague a few days after his return for a holiday. "Hi, I haven't seen you for ages, mate. Have you been working down The Annex?" That was really what it was like - being in another country on the opposite side of the world!

However, this particular ward that I was allocated to work in was small and cosy, housing a similar group of elderly white-haired ladies as seen in my previous experience. One of my memories from this ward was working with an older Irish 'made up' SEN who seemed very frightened and threatened that maybe we students might have some more knowledge than her, having experienced some formal training in the School of Nursing.

I have already mentioned some assistant nurses being promoted to State Enrolled Nurses many years ago if they had years of experience, as there was a serious shortage of qualified nurses, but sadly some of these were promoted without the backup of a solid knowledge base or any training. Usually they were second in command to a registered staff nurse or sister, but not always.

This particular nurse liked to show her authority by saying she was in charge and holding the keys to everything, but when I worked with her, she had me doing all the medicine rounds, dressings and dealing with any medic who might come to the ward to assess a patient who may have become quite poorly. She seemed to disappear into a side room and literally pushed me into the office to deal with anything 'medical'. However, when the coast was clear and the doctor had gone, she would appear to interrogate me to put her in the picture as to what needed to be done. It provided an excellent experience for me as a student, but I know she felt totally out of her depth, and it was sad that she couldn't be more honest about how she felt. It was pretty obvious that she was anxious and worried about being asked about something she didn't know. There is just nothing wrong with saying, "I don't know", as it is often a chance to learn something new!

Another memory from that ward was that our kitchen door faced a main corridor in the annex and often other patients wandering up and down would sneak into our kitchen and steal food or even take a bite out of something left on the worktop. I often hid watching them and let them get away with it, as regular ward staff knew about it, saying it was probably a response from past days when all food was dished out at a set time by a nurse in charge and there was no way of getting more or a snack in between meals if you were hungry. Also, they daren't ask for more in those days, as the rules were strictly abided by. It put me in mind of Dickens's Oliver in another Victorian institution. It takes some courage to steal and swallow a whole piece of cake in two seconds and then continue walking down the corridor innocently, as many did. These were often male patients from another ward who probably had a larger appetite and felt hungry.

Some of the older staff on that ward seemed just as institutionalised as the patients. They had worked for many years down the annex, where everybody knew everybody, so we student interlopers were to be sometimes viewed with suspicion and had to tread carefully to be accepted. You felt like an outsider and had to prove you could be trusted!

There were rumours that one sister ran a catalogue club and sold items to patients, making commission on her sales. Or there was a married couple of trained nurses who had furnished their house with hospital items and had regular coal and meat deliveries from hospital supplies. I heard a male nurse say he was invited by the husband to their house for a drink after work one day. He said he sat back and looked around and suddenly felt a sense of deja vu, as he thought he was back at work in the hospital because their furniture, carpet and curtains were very familiar!

Then there were those who ate patients' food, smoked patients' cigarettes and helped themselves to hospital supplies as they wanted. I like to feel these were a minority of staff, and thankfully these practices became less easy to hide as change came, with an opening up of secret cupboards and minds! Remembering that staff were there to care for the patients, not to help themselves, and these practices were strictly forbidden and illegal. But when some of those in charge are corrupt, who do you report it to?

Saying all this, there were lovely older staff too, such as one Italian nurse who would make large tray pizzas on a Sunday afternoon for staff and patients or another who would make delicious potato cakes out of leftover mashed potato, of which there was always plenty. Some of the old wards smelt of mashed potato. Then sometimes patients would have a drug-free Sunday, and they would get a bottle of stout or a tot of sherry if they wanted for a treat. This was not prescribed but usually directed at the discretion of the nurse in charge. Much of their medication was of a tranquilliser or sedative nature, and consumption over a long period of time would either create a tolerance to the drug when the patient doesn't feel any benefit from it, or it may build up in the body and create very sleepy, sedated individuals who didn't move much or get much out of life. Small drug holidays were probably a beneficial thing.

On this ward there was an older German domestic who was a young adult during the Second World War. She told stories of living in Dresden in Germany when it was heavily bombed. She described going out dancing and returning in the early hours to find her home and family gone in a pile of rubble, of sleeping in the street, being hungry and walking for days in high-heeled shoes lopsided with one heel missing until some help became available for all those victims of bombing. She was always very kind and loving to all the patients and very grateful for her life in England, saying she had experienced a horrendous side of life as a young woman, seeing things she would never forget. People who have had difficult times in life can often be very helpful, empathetic and understanding to others who are also experiencing difficulties.

Talking about the effects of war, there were many patients still in the hospital in the 1970s who were emotional casualties from the Second World War. We call this Post Traumatic Stress Disorder now, hopefully understanding that this condition is very serious and debilitating but can be treated and does not warrant staying in a large mental hospital for 20 plus years anymore. During their war experiences in the past, some had a diagnosis of 'Shell Shock' or were seen as cowards and executed just because they had a total mental breakdown and maybe ran away or exhibited strange behaviour. During war the noise, filth, blood, disgusting mutilation of bodies and death are enough to disturb most humans. Thankfully we are more understanding and informed nowadays. Yet wars still continue in the world today, and as a human race we continue to destroy, maim and kill each other, leaving many victims of war emotionally scarred and changed forever. Why don't we ever learn?

All long stay patients were given a small allowance of money each week for personal items or treats. So it was a job, usually at the weekend when the ward was quieter, to complete the 'patients' parcels order book', which involved talking with each patient and asking them what they would like to spend their money on. Some were talkative and wanted cigs, toiletries, tins of fruit or chocolate, but others didn't talk much or at all and didn't know or say what they wanted. They hadn't spent money on themselves for years and had forgotten how to choose or want anything. As a result, when it was my turn to complete this book, I tried to order items on their behalf, knowing a little about them, having worked with them over a period of time, if they were not very forthcoming with any suggestions or ideas.

I never felt very comfortable with this, choosing for someone, but staff were advised to spend this allowance and not really encourage letting this money build up in the 'patients; affairs department'. The fear being, as with most government funding, that it would be taken away if not used and considered to be needed. So bathroom toiletries were purchased and used for all, despite having individual names written on them. Tights and stockings were bought for women and shaving toiletries for men. Sweets, chocolates and tinned items were also ordered. These items were all bought at the hospital shop, so I presume the money automatically went back into the system. So an individual patient didn't really have a chance to manage their own money or save. The institution remained in charge.

Also, if you were lucky enough to get inside some of the secret cupboards on some of the long stay wards, you would find a very well-stocked cave of items which had built up over time.

So when the nurse in charge (the key holder) was away, I always made sure the patients had plenty of treats as we raided the cupboard. Oh yes, party time! But one memory stays with me of working on one of these wards where we normally made sandwiches for all the patients for their tea, as they always had a cooked dinner at midday. The kitchen would send salad, cheese and cooked meat to make these sandwiches, but sometimes we would use for individual patients an item from their treats. Some liked tuna sandwiches or tinned fruit and cream as a treat.

On this particular occasion, I made sandwiches with a tin of tuna for a particular patient and put her name on them. Nobody had told me that she was very fussy and normally had her tuna just tipped onto a plate with bread and butter on the side. So when she saw what I had done, she had a tantrum, gave me plenty of abuse despite my apologies and scraped every bit of tuna off my sandwiches, shaped it into a round and then proceeded to eat it by putting it back on the bread herself.

I felt really awful, but the regular staff just said, "Ignore her; she has a typical epileptic personality." I asked, "What is an epileptic personality?" The staff nurse said, "Well, years ago, epilepsy was misunderstood, and even now the public are alarmed if they see someone have a seizure. The person can foam at the mouth or become incontinent, and years ago this was considered to be true madness. So many people who suffered seizures were shunned and rejected, causing many to have a 'chip on their shoulder', feeling that they were persecuted by everyone, which, due to ignorance, was probably quite true." It seems to be human nature to steer clear of something you don't understand.

Most people who have never seen somebody have a fit are often quite alarmed by it and don't know what to do. The sufferer also feels embarrassed, especially if they have wet themselves during the fit or dribbled uncontrollably in front of all their colleagues or friends. Also years ago there wasn't the medication we have now to help control seizures. Sadly, due to ignorance, many of these long stay patients were in the hospital for years and years mainly just because they suffered from epilepsy or may have reacted badly to others not understanding.

That lady never spoke to me again after the tuna incident despite my efforts to seek forgiveness. I felt this incident gave me some insight and helped me to understand what this 'epileptic personality' theory was about, for many good reasons, although there is no scientific evidence for judging or labelling anyone in that way. Thank goodness we now have more information and medication to control fits so that many can lead a fairly normal life in the community. As with many conditions, ignorance and prejudice have caused all sorts of problems. It is just sad that some of those long stay patients were often there for many years just because they had epilepsy and staff referred to some wards as epileptic wards. All the more reason for change!

NIGHT DUTY

During our training both Debbi and I spent a compulsory period of twelve weeks on 'nights'. Night duty was not a rotational thing as in some hospitals, but at that time in our hospital there were permanent night staff and day staff and sometimes a fair bit of competition between the two. In saying that, I mean often blaming each other for things not done properly or probably not understanding each other's world, so as we all know, ignorance often can breed false ideas and bad feelings.

The fact that students had to spend three months on night duty as part of their training was a good way for them to see how the 'night world' functioned. Some staff had been on permanent night duty for many years and loved it, whereas it just didn't suit some people who couldn't get into a sleep pattern and felt dreadful throughout. In my opinion it was a different world, which of course is quite normal, because even at home our own behaviour changes in the evening as we prepare for sleep, and so did the patients' whom we were looking after. Being tired or unable to sleep can produce another whole raft of mental health problems. Insomnia can often be one of the first symptoms of the start of a mental health breakdown.

Once on duty at 7:00pm, a 'brew' was usually consumed whilst the day staff nurse in charge would do the handover, updating the night staff on the day's events and each patient's progress. This would vary depending on the ward, as not much changed on some long stay wards, yet things moved dramatically on admission wards sometimes. So some of the staff who worked on long stay wards on nights worked alone and were mainly caretakers to be there just in case there was a problem. There were tales of some of these staff who had been there for many years and fitted in very well at the asylum, as they had their own strange behaviours and didn't really socially interact with anyone in or out of work. Some lived in the nurses' home so long that they had become part of the institution. For some this was a very safe, unchanging environment for a long time, so when change came along, many of these staff couldn't cope.

On the other hand, working on a busy admission ward could be a challenge for just one qualified nurse and a student or nursing assistant, especially if someone was disturbed or a new emergency admission came in during the night. The individual could be noisy, angry, wanting to fight and would most definitely be upset, frightened and not wanting to be there. However, some might be subdued, mute or glad to feel they were in a safe place. A whole mix of skills would be needed by the nurse in these situations. A good measure is always how I would feel if it was me and what kind of help I would want. It is very important to give people information and be honest so they can trust you and understand what is going to happen. So hopefully that will reduce any fear, preventing possible violence.

During our training we attended courses and updates on how to deal with a violent or difficult situation and suggestions like wrapping someone in a blanket to restrain them or learning various blocking techniques, which were all well and good, but when someone is heading for you like a roaring bull, it sometimes is every man for himself. That is run, hide and lock yourself in or out.

Thankfully those situations, as I said previously, were very rare. The more you worked with people with mental health problems, the more you realised that it is often the so-called sane ones in the outside world that you need to fear.

Those staff on nights had a large social network, and many would visit each other on their breaks during the night. Sometimes the police would call in for a chat and a brew. One nurse had regular visits from different staff, as she saw herself as a clairvoyant. There was much knitting, playing card games, reading, even crown green bowling on the large dayroom carpets and some secret parties! All this activity seemed to help the long night pass by. It felt like one big social club. Patients were cared for, and staff were generally happy on the whole.

The wards were a bit eerie at night with long dark corridors, but as the patients slept and all was quiet at night in the old buildings with low lighting, sometimes mice would come out quite tamely, as some nurses used to feed them. My experiences on nights were enjoyable in that I met many interesting people, learned to deal with all sorts of situations alone and found most of the staff a happy, friendly lot with a great sense of humour. The whole atmosphere was more laidback at night, and as a nurse on the ward, you had the time to sit and chat during the evening or night if a patient was having difficulty getting to sleep. So we would sometimes pull up an armchair, make them a hot drink and wrap them in a blanket. We chatted about everyday things, getting to know them a little better, which was sometimes more difficult during the day when there was less time with so much more to do, and before you knew it, they had dozed off in the armchair. Result!

One of the worst things was when the police brought somebody in, quite disturbed, frightened, maybe fighting or shouting, and in those days, in my experience, the police didn't have many skills to diffuse the situation. So often two nurses were left alone to deal with the individual until a doctor arrived to prescribe some calming medication if needed. That was the time to learn how to try and diffuse a very tense situation. Can you imagine being agitated, lost, frightened or upset and being manhandled into a police van and then dropped off at a psychiatric ward? It is enough to make anyone panic and come out shouting and fighting. Most people's reaction when presented with someone 'in an aggressive state' is to run for your life or try to take control by confronting it with more aggression.

Quite honestly, in all the years I worked in the job, most very disturbed patients responded well to you backing off, trying to relax, and showing kindness and understanding, which is what we all respond to, but on a few occasions the job was to contain someone to make them and others safe until the situation had calmed down. I have wrestled on the floor with people or sat astride them very occasionally, but that was very rare. I am glad, very glad, to say.

It was always important to try to remain calm, speaking slowly and quietly but firmly. Give as much reassurance as possible and try to be friendly, letting the person know you are on their side and are there to try and help. Fear makes us all behave in a crazy manner!

When someone is severely psychotic, anxious or paranoid, they can behave really aggressively towards you as a nurse, saying and threatening all kinds of things, but as they receive treatment and start to feel better, they often apologise for the things they said or did at that time. I have had that happen to me on several occasions.

One of the skills you try to learn with experience is how to distinguish between the mad and the bad. Even then you don't always get it right, as some will think they are allowed to behave badly on a psychiatric ward and mask symptoms to get what they want or get away with something bad that they have done. However, in time with observation, these individuals usually become exposed and are discharged.

Some of Debbi's night duty experiences were as follows: Predominantly the night staff had been working there for many, many years, and this was not dissimilar to my first ward experience previously discussed, an elderly female long stay ward, but I was not quite so naive by then. As soon as the day staff left at 7:00pm, it was time to start 'winding the patients down'. We were allowed to sit and interact with the ladies on the ward, and I found this was actually a good time, as mostly they were tired from their pacing all day, and many wanted to sit and even fall asleep in their chairs. But no! Rules and routines must be followed at all times! Supper consisted of more weak tea in the giant teapots, but also the same scratchy pots offered what was described as cocoa. Ugh, it looked vile; again, sugar was added before pouring, and I can only describe the colour as dirty milk. It did not matter if you stirred it from the bottom; it still resembled dishwater. Biscuits too were on offer, two per patient and no more. I witnessed many with 'a cunning plan' to steal from others or fight for an extra biscuit. There were also many examples of favouritism when three or even four stuck together and were very quickly pushed into hungry, often toothless mouths and washed down with the dishwater.

Something that sticks in my mind was the medication rounds at night. Nobody was told to come and get their medication; there was always a queue. I guess bedtime was the most exciting time of the day. The medication offered some oblivion.

Staff would go into the dormitories with the ladies, as some needed help to undress, others just needed encouragement to remove day clothes and put on one of the bum-flashing nighties, and then they would attempt to get between the tight sheets and get warm. At home we still had blankets on the beds, but if it was cold, Mum would give us another one, and I remember the lovely feeling of the extra weight of an extra blanket. The dormitory-style rooms with approx. four feet between the beds were always cold and unwelcoming. There were no pictures on the walls that I can remember, no cupboards or shelves, just the beds. I also remember the dorms being quite echoey. Sadly it was a sheet and a cotton counterpane. I am not sure when it happened, but I do remember cotton blankets with holes in were also introduced. I honestly don't think anybody in the hospital will be remembering the comforting feeling of that extra warm and heavy blanket, sadly!

More often than not they lay there as if they had been strapped in, unable to move. I remember thinking the nighties must ride up and split open as they tried to wriggle down the tight bedding. How uncomfortable!

You will not believe what I will tell you next, but I swear to you it is true; it was as bad as I will describe and also a common night initiation practice!

When the staff (all unqualified; there was one qualified for four wards each night, and he/she moved between them to do a drug round and monitor) settled in the office with their knitting (yes, knitting), I was told to go into the day room and switch off the lights. There were approx. 10-12 switches on large boards; it was a big room. There was low lighting to the corridor leading to the dormitories at the far end of the room. I went to do some jobs, clearing up in the kitchen and doing some 'bundles'. I also sat with the staff and chewed the fat! After about two hours I was told to go to the dormitories and do a check. I was told to "put one set of lights on so you don't trip over the tables." Well, I did… Oh my Lord, I have never seen anything like it!

As I stepped into the room with one hand going up to the lights, I was aware of movement on the floor; the previously coloured carpet was black and moving! There was a low clicking sort of noise, and I realised I was standing on a carpet of enormous cockroaches! Thousands of them! They quickly moved like the sea parting and disappeared under the skirting boards! Ugh, it was horrible as well as fascinating. I heard laughing behind me and realised I had been had! What did I learn? Don't switch off the lights at night!

Truthfully I cannot describe what it looked like. I had seen lots of cockroaches in Wards 1 and 2 before, even in the kitchen. I opened a drawer, and one ran up my arm! But this nightly carpet was unbelievable.

En route to the canteen during the night, I would walk through the kitchens, and many times I saw the kitchen staff whacking the cockroaches with heavy implements, but they would still get up and run away underneath a piece of equipment. Ugh, horrible crawly creatures. The wards at night were very eerie, generally quiet, and then suddenly you would hear an ear-piercing scream or a shout, or loud swearing. Sadly, those poor people suffered the demons at night as well.

Night shifts for me were hard; as I said previously, I liked my sleep, and sleeping in the nurses' home was not easy. There was always someone selfish who would knock on your door and run away, despite the sign on the door stating, 'ON NIGHTS,

GO AWAY!' There was very little learning going on either. The wards were staffed with auxiliary staff who had been around a very long time, and although generally they cared about the patients, routines were very much the order of the night. Breaks were long and gossip rife! And so much knitting! Everyone seemed to knit and smoke.

The canteen at night was quite an experience; as I was to learn later, it was an extension of the social club! After drinking all evening, people would go to the canteen for food before heading home, having a short sleep and going back to work to start at 7:00am.

You have probably gathered I avoided nights as often as I could; in fact, if I recall, I did those three months and a few overtime shifts when I needed extra cash, and that was pretty much it, thank goodness.

We have both recounted our night duty experiences, which were very similar, probably due to the fact that nothing much changed and night duty remained constant for years. Following our night duty experiences, needless to say, neither of us ever worked the night shifts again. Although it was an important experience to have, we have both noted that it was an experience we rarely shared. Unlike daytime experiences, permanent night workers would probably say different; that was their world and not ours.

PHYSICAL CARE

Another type of experience during our training was to work on a physical care ward. As we all do, those with mental health problems suffer with physical illnesses too. This ward that I, Angela, worked on within the psychiatric hospital was staffed by many general nursing-trained staff nurses, and it was where I learned so much more about the more physical care of a patient. However, Debbi went to work in a local general hospital to receive her physical health care experience and came face to face with the general public, whereas I cared for those who had a psychiatric condition but had become physically unwell.

It was hilarious at times when you have a treatment plan for a certain physical condition, but a patient whose mind is disturbed, confused or depressed doesn't always listen to instructions or understand what you are saying. So it was quite a challenge in many ways to succeed in offering the right treatment or care.

For instance, we had an outbreak of Salmonella, a very contagious stomach bug. So we had half the ward segregated and were barrier nursing some of the patients who had tested positive. Now Walter, who had been in the hospital many years, didn't ever speak but could hear, just didn't get why he was to stay in a restricted part of the ward, so he regularly ran up and down the ward and got in any bed that he fancied, even if there was somebody else in it.

So as nurses we had to 'gown up', i.e. wear protective clothing and masks, to enter the restricted area of the ward, where patients were infectious, just as they have had to do during the recent Covid epidemic. So chasing after this particular patient meant getting dressed and undressed in the middle of the ward very quickly, like in an old silent movie, which reduced us to laughter in the end. As a result, someone had to stand guard at the screens dividing the ward and send Walter back to his own bed every time he fancied a wander.

Needless to say, we were very happy and relieved when he had three clear stool results and was sent back to his own ward.

I learnt how to deal with infusions and suction machines and assist in minor operations, as there was a small operating theatre attached to this ward for use by the general public, which we staffed for some reason. We also helped with anaesthesia and recovery. The generally trained nurses were used to patients who could be trusted to take their own medication and follow instructions like "Don't get out of bed and try to walk" or "Don't take the bandage off", but our patients often didn't do as you hoped, so much more supervision was needed. That was why if one of our patients was poorly enough to be transferred to a general hospital, one of our mental health nurses had to go with them to 'special' them, which meant sitting with them and caring for their every need, as they couldn't be trusted to be left alone or could be at risk in some way.

Many of the general nurses in the General Hospital kept well away. Probably part of the fear and misunderstanding that the general public have of mental health problems. Sad that some of that still exists even now. It is a more recognised fact now that our mental health plays a huge part in our physical health. The two just can't be separated, as a positive mental state aids a good physical outcome, or even a positive mental attitude aids coping with the symptoms.

DEBBI'S PHYSICAL CARE EXPERIENCE

As Debbi has previously said, she had to spend 12 whole weeks on a general hospital ward. This is how she recalls her experience.

I was sent to a female orthopaedic ward, and I had to live in the nurses' home there, which was horrible. Nobody was friendly, lights out at 10:00pm, and I recall no laughter, and everything was always tense somehow. Looking back I probably brought it on myself and was distant and made it clear I did not want to be there. The ward sister was unbelievably out of touch with the rest of the world in my view; we really did not hit it off. It was as if she wanted complete control; nobody could speak to her, she was unapproachable, and everything was non-negotiable. She demonstrated no compassion for the patients on the ward; she never smiled or lightened the mood, ever.

I recall her asking me if I knew how to take a temperature and blood pressure and count respirations. I was so insulted; I was wearing a uniform for goodness sake! So I said NO. I then allowed a poor nurse to teach me again! The Witch, as I fondly named her in my head, wasn't stupid; she said I had to wear a red belt to identify me from the general nursing students, so I wrote 'FROM the LUNATIC ASYLUM' on my hat the next day, and she was apoplectic! So funny, I can still see her face now, hehehe. She pulled it off my head and sent me to the sluice all day. Witch! She then reported me to the nursing officer at my lovely, wonderful hospital, and I was sent back to be disciplined. Really, unbeknown to the Witch, that nursing officer was a wonderful, kind, understanding, generous and wise man who said, "What the hell have you been doing now? Go back and tell her you have had a bollocking and keep your head down for once in your life!"

That man was to become a lifelong friend and a very important person to me and my family in so many ways. He was a remarkable man, and he married my best friend, eventually!

So it was back to the Witch ward for me ... A young Canadian girl, in the UK on holiday, was admitted with a broken back following a car accident, bless her. I still remember her distress. She was to be flat on her back for many weeks. I took it upon myself to wash her lovely long blonde hair one day before she went for an X-ray (she had told me she fancied the young porter, and why not give her an opportunity to have some fun, eh?). Well, her head was hanging over the back of the bed and a bucket in place to catch the water, hair wet and about to be lathered, and in walked the Witch. "What do you think you are doing?", "Washing her hair," was my reply. "Not today you are not!" There was no good reason given; I had nothing else to do, and of course the other patients on the ward were watching and listening, which she was aware of. I carried on, and you should have seen her face! I knew I was in big trouble, but what the hell, she went for her X-ray with shiny hair. Unfortunately it wasn't the young porter who collected her, but that was ok.

One other great memory from the Witch ward that I want to share with you was when I told the patients (men and women in those days on the same ward) that before the end of my shift they would see the Witch's knickers. It caused great excitement and giggles. Some of the other nurses seemed to like me, probably because I challenged the stupid woman and her ridiculous rules. Anyway, that afternoon was the ward round. The Witch, the consultant and all his entourage of junior doctors, etc., entered the ward (I was in the sluice as usual just in case I caused trouble). She pushed a steel trolley with all the files on it from bed to bed where they spoke to each other, not to the patient, by the way! And then, right on cue, a planned pee bottle was needed by the chap at the bottom of the ward. Off I went, scurrying like the maid I was, and oh no! I knocked the trolley with the files on! Argh! They fell to the floor, and the poor witch had to bend down to pick them up! Knickers on full display, hahaha, so funny, the patients actually clapped and laughed out loud. She should follow her own rules and wear her uniform at the correct length and not like something out of a Carry On film!

Needless to say, I was in big trouble again! Off I was sent! "I never want to see you anywhere near my ward again."

Of course I failed the placement, but the sensible staff at the 'asylum', although they were a bit dismayed, gave me the opportunity to be assessed on the physical ward at our hospital, and of course I was perfectly competent to reach the required standard and passed the module, haha. But with only two weeks of my 12 to go, I had a week's holiday and a week on the medical ward at the asylum, and I was freed... hooray. I most definitely could not be a nurse in a general hospital.

You may note I am at this point still using the word 'asylum'; that is what it was referred to as, but times were beginning to change, and there was talk of massive changes on the horizon in mental health care, including the law. The *1959 Mental Health Act*{1} was being challenged. It was originally designed to repeal the *1890 Lunacy Act*{3} and the *1930 Mental Health Act*{4}; and to make way for the treatment and care of mentally disordered individuals away from institutionalised care and into the community. Being a part of this bigger plan was very exciting, and it allowed me (us) to challenge some of the archaic practices that were no longer needed and did not move along with the improvement in scientific knowledge and subsequently better treatments, both pharmacological and psychological.

So back to the Asylum... you know, using that word, 'Asylum', feels disrespectful now, but then that is what it was called. It became the hospital at some point in my career, which I guess is an improvement, but the mental health services soon became psychiatric 'wings' of general hospitals, and the closure of the large asylums was imminent. I often wonder about that young Canadian girl and hope she got home to her family and lived a good life. I never think about the Witch, but I do think about what I learned through that experience, and never did I treat junior staff like she did. All staff of all grades are learning every day; we learn from each other and everyone has something to contribute. You get far more from people who are happy in work, appreciated and respected.

THE BIG MOVE FOR DEBBI

I had had enough of working 12–15 hour shifts and getting a bus back to my house share. My non-nursing housemates worked normal hours and lived normal lives. As I was getting home exhausted, they were going out to have fun, and then they would come in late and wake me, and I would disturb them in the early morning too. I was moving into the nurses' home!

Don't misunderstand me; the reasons above were very genuine and I was very grateful to my cousin for enabling me to make a massive step in my life. But… it was time to move on. I had been to see friends in the nurses' home, and I really liked it; there was always someone about, and it felt so grown up and fun!

The room I had been allocated was in the older of the two homes, not refurbished like the other option, but the rooms were bigger, and the housekeeper (one very scary lady) preferred to spend more time in the refurbed, or so the story went. I was allocated an amazing room! It was large, and a big sash window that had been painted so many times was difficult to open (I would sort that out) and overlooked the lovely, well-kept grounds and cricket pitch. Below me was THE SOCIAL CLUB! 10 strides and I was going down the back steps to the club. I thought I had died and gone to heaven! No more late-night buses with dodgy characters on board, no more early-morning bus stops waiting to see the milkman who flashed at me - not his lights, by the way! He frequently dropped his pants and made lewd comments. I told him I would tell the police, but it made no difference, so I just used to say things like "Put it away, or it will drop off" or "See the uniform, mate? I have seen more of those than you have had hot dinners," or if I felt really cruel… suffice to say I would comment on his lack of size! Good god! Today I would be appalled and wouldn't hesitate to go to the police.

Don't forget that times were very different back then. I am not saying it was ok, because it was not, but at the end of the day

I truly believe people were not only more tolerant, but much more resilient emotionally. I could not go home and search the internet, and neither did I hear of the potential difficulties which could arise if the 'flasher' was not stopped and how his behaviour could escalate to something much more serious. I couldn't go on Facebook and tell the world; I just got on with it. Today, young people do not need to develop coping skills in difficult situations. Don't misunderstand me; I could talk to friends and colleagues, and if I was frightened, I would have had lots of support, but to be honest, it was just a life event and it didn't bother me.

Anyway, back to the big move. Mum and Dad helped out again, of course. They moved me in and bought all sorts of things, from nice mugs to a rug and a plant, and I remember a macrame hanger. For those who haven't a clue what the latter item is – it is a stringy crochet-type thing for hanging plants, pots or coloured glass balls or anything, actually. Very 'cool' in the '70s. Everybody had one.

Dad brought tools, of course! He always has half the garage to hand! He fixed the window so it opened freely, mended the curtain rail and refitted the curtains which were hanging off. I remember I had to go looking for a ladder because the windows were huge and very high. I left Dad to this and took Mum on a tour of my new home. Two floors, mine on the top floor, creaking old and uneven floors and stairs led down a corridor with blue highly glossed doors on the left, a telephone booth on the corner (which I was able to hear from my room with the door open if I was expecting a call), a small kitchen which would allow for making a snack or hot drinks, and two communal fridges and kettles. Shower and bathrooms, which I remember my mum saying, "need a damned good clean". The housekeeper would have had a fit! I shall call her H for now. I recall deliberately not telling Mum and Dad how close I was to the social club! No need to worry the parents eh! Dad was still not comfortable with me being in the hospital at all, but by now I think he knew I was not going home. They seemed reassured by H, who came to my room to meet them and to tell them about all the strict rules relating to no men in your room, silence after 10.00, and no guests (but I could book the spare room for a guest occasionally; my younger brother came once but only once. I think we walked through the corridors from the club to the canteen at night, and he did not like it!). Also no alcohol, no pets, and definitely no parties. It seems nobody read the rule book, though! Much of what went on in the nurses' home shall remain a secret!

There was a communal lounge area, a big room with huge, battered leather sofas, and I remember the heating pipes running along the floor, which were massive! Which was why my first domestic-type purchase was a wooden clothes maiden to dry my washing (there was no such thing as a tumble dryer, believe it or not!), which joined the rest of the clothes maidens in the lounge, and we all lounged in each other's rooms! As for gatherings, they happened every day and every night, depending on whether you were on night or day shift. Pets – my neighbour had a parrot! Someone else, a rat, and well, eventually I acquired a dog! Again, another story, but suffice to say that I pushed the boundaries and eventually I was 'asked to leave', but that was a long time after my first day there.

When I think back and draw comparisons with my sons and their experience of leaving the nest, I had (or needed) very little in terms of 'stuff'. We were all in the same boat, broke most of the time and very tired from studying and working 12-hour shifts, but we were all very positive and happy.

When our eldest went to the USA, he needed everything: laptop, games console, and even a car eventually! Student accommodation there was luxury and even included a BBQ and pool. However, he too worked hard and played hard, as part of growing up and mapping out your life, I guess. We used to say he survived the USA champagne lifestyle on lager money! Bless him!

University in the UK for our youngest was a bit more modest but laptop, mobile and yes… eventually a car! But my argument for that was in order for him to get home! Haha.

I had my room, my plant, my precious books, and I thought I was really spoilt, as I even had a hairdryer… of my own! It was a magical time of my life.

I soon got sick of people stealing things from the fridge, milk and cheese being about the only things I kept there. My dad suggested I put a label on stating I HAVE SPAT IN THIS. Guess what? It worked. Haha. Well done, Dad.

The luxury of getting up 15 minutes before starting a shift was amazing! Up, wash, out. 12 hours later, in and change, then social club! That was a very vibrant place; lots of beer, weed, and music. There was a dance floor in the middle, and seemingly it did not matter what time of day it was; there were folks there drinking and dancing. Maybe they had worked all night or even went in for a couple of pints before their shift (yes, this is actually true!).

It was here that my and Angela's friendship blossomed. I had been befriended by the cool guy in the Afghan coat, previously mentioned by Angela! He was obviously very friendly with her too! We spent a lot of time together, and my love for them and their tribe of boys developed at a rapid rate and I was adopted into their family eventually; there was no going back!

QUALIFIED AT LAST

We think and talk about the changes now, and thus far we have both shared some of our memorable experiences of the time, probably memorable now because we both find it hard to believe that we were a part of some of the practices, and the difficult lives those people led in the institution that was there to care for them. Was it as difficult for some as living in communities where they were vulnerable and ridiculed and misunderstood? There was also a lot of care and thoughtfulness and love behind those walls, and sadly, not all the changes were for the good. Maybe we will come to that later.

Nevertheless, before that I had to qualify as a nurse… and get myself kicked out of the nurses' home. Exams were never good for me; I hated them in school, and I hated them during my training. Even if I worked hard and felt confident, nerves would always get the better of me. I was later on very grateful to acquire some good advice from a charge nurse who had qualified a few years before. He said always imagine the person reading your answers knows nothing about psychiatry, nursing or mental illness, and you have to make sure you tell them everything you know. Don't assume they know. So I did just that. I still remember the *1959 Mental Health Act*{1} now, as I learned it like a parrot.

My wonderful friend, who is writing alongside me, somehow found out the night before results day who had passed, something to do with our papers being marked in Birmingham or something. I really don't know, but she asked me, "Do you want to know?" I said "Yes", and then the party started! Mum and Dad were cross with me for finding out early and said I should wait until the next morning, but what they didn't know wouldn't hurt them, is what I thought!

I recall being put in the shower by (yes, you again, my friend) only to be dressed and back down the steps to the social club. We danced and sang and got very, very drunk. The next morning I found all my underwear from my room hanging from a tree outside. Mortified, I was! And I never did find out who had done it. That was the type of thing we used to do to each other, just for laughs. When I think of some of the states I have turned up on the ward in and completed a 12-hour shift. Now it makes my toes curl, but then… well, it was the done thing! The best one was daring to hang the matron's knickers from the clock tower! I am pretty sure they were not Matron's big knickers, but they were definitely large and definitely hanging from the small hand of the clock one morning to greet everyone coming in for the 7.00 am shift. Haha. Not me, I hasten to add, way too high, but I did stand guard while the knickers were nicked from the laundry!

DEBBI - EVER THE RULE BREAKER

I was told about a dog rescue centre a few miles away, and myself and two others decided we would go and see it. Why? Who knows! But we did, and they had a Saturday cage; basically, this meant that if a dog was in a Saturday cage, it would be put to sleep that day. It must have been a Friday when we went, because I came home with a black Lab cross puppy.

Oh yes, my friends said they would help, and we would be able to hide her from the housekeeper at all times. We lasted three months! Did well, really, I think, and then my notice to leave was final. NO PETS AND NO BOYFRIENDS. Apparently I knew the rules, so out you go!

Of course I was so in love with my Tessa by then; she was my pal, my soulmate. When I wasn't working, she came everywhere with me. I had a car at this point (thanks, Mum and Dad), and she used to lie on the back window of my Austin 1100, wherever I went. She used to come to the pub, and along with my pint, I was always given a clean ashtray with water in for her. She was so spoilt by everyone. The longer-term solution was to take her home to Mum and Dad, but that just didn't seem to happen; she stayed with me and had a very happy life.

It wasn't hard to find somewhere to live; most people were associated with the hospital in one way or another, and I shared a house with friends, three of us. We had a garden for Tessa and so much fun! Of course I was seriously grown up by then, wasn't I?

I recall earning £136.00 per month, but then I had to find rent and money for bills, which was tough, to be honest, but we were all in the same boat, and we could make a loaf of bread last a long time!

I recall my car breaking down, as it needed a new water pump. Cue Dad again! I got a lift to a scrapyard to buy a water pump and decided I really could take the old one off and put a 'new' one on. Don't forget we had no YouTube, mobile phones, or Automobile Roadside Assistance in those days (well, there probably was an AA service, but I certainly could not have afforded it if there had been), so this job was completed one hot sunny Sunday, with me going into the house for instructions from Dad on the phone and back outside to do a bit, then back into the house for more instructions. I even made a new gasket. I think it was cardboard. I don't really remember, but it involved drawing around the old water pump and cutting it out before fixing it to the pump and main body of the engine. It worked too! I am not sure of the relevance of that memory, really, but I think it was stirred by thoughts of change and how our lives are so different now in many, many ways, some for the better but sadly, not all.

I did meet many, many very lonely individuals recently during my work, and this is the thing I struggle with most. I have, as I said previously, truly believed that recovery is possible, but, to achieve this, we have to allow individuals to express what recovery is for them, not for us.

Unfortunately I do not believe we are quite there all the time because today's service has removed the social opportunities that were naturally available in the asylums: mixing with like-minded people, having a role, having aspirations (even if those aspirations were only to get to the bible to remove the best pages to roll leftover tobacco out of the 'dimps' before someone else!). I am not trying to make light of this, but social inclusion is very difficult to achieve if it is offered by a service that believes they know what is best. This is what happens all too often: services are so strapped for cash all they can manage is to pay lip service to the concept of social inclusion and recovery. It seems that if an individual feels that recovery for him/her is to remain in a service-run drop-in group, why then do we feel so uncomfortable when it appears this may be forever needed by that individual?

I have moved ahead too quickly here, maybe a sign of how strongly I feel about it!

ONWARDS AND UPWARDS AS QUALIFIED NURSES

Well, I did it – I became a qualified mental health nurse! I had a career, and I was very ambitious and desperate to be the best!

I secured a job as a staff nurse on the adolescent unit, a new modern building in the grounds (albeit on the edge) of the main hospital. No more uniforms; we were given a mufti allowance to help towards clothing costs. It wasn't much, but I guess it helped.

I think it is important to say at this point that (and I can only give my personal opinion) the need to ensure that the young people on the unit, who were really very disturbed individuals aged between 11 and 16, had a very different experience of mental health services. There was a determination that these individuals never experience the service delivered to the folks in the main hospital. As I have suggested, it was a time of massive change, and I was very privileged to be part of it. My time on the unit laid the foundations for my future career. I was able to voice an opinion and be heard. Although there was a hierarchy, all staff worked together, and we worked alongside the young people. We shared skills and knowledge and valued each other's opinions. Every staff member on the team was dedicated to improving outcomes for the youngsters in our care.

As a junior member of staff who had just left training, I was so excited and determined until one day I went to open the door (which was locked) to greet visitors for one of the kids, and I was asked, "Can you tell us where we can find a member of staff, please?" I was gutted, imagine! They thought I was one of the kids! I explained I was a staff nurse, and they, and my colleagues, also thought it was funny! Haha, no harm done, and I was quite young!

We had rotas for jobs on the unit, and though I was ok with the cooking rota, it was sometimes difficult gauging how much food to prepare. The kids were on the rota too, and predominantly they chose what to cook. I reckon they had better preparation for the real world than youngsters who were in mainstream school in the community.

Supporting the kids to keep their rooms clean and tidy(ish) was the one I did not like particularly, mainly because some of the kids had belongings and 'stuff' that showed they had families and others who cared about them and were waiting for them to go home, whereas others had nothing, few clothes, no photos, and nobody waiting for them to go home. Hearing the backgrounds and difficulties which led to their arrival on the unit from anywhere in the country was often harrowing.

I think I have locked away many of the things I witnessed, as it was difficult to hear, but I do have lasting memories of good and important times, and I am mindful that if our memories are ever read by anyone other than my wonderful friend and me, some of those young people might read and remember the time they spent on the unit trying to help each other through some very difficult times.

One very strong and positive memory, however, was taking a group on a camping trip to Wales to 'avoid the royal wedding'! I recall the comments and faces of some kids who had never been anywhere like it before. Part of me felt guilty that I could enjoy the peace, the quiet and the outside world whenever I chose to, really. To this day I like to believe that that trip gave them some hope and the opportunity to realise that life could take a different direction for them if only they could be strong and optimistic and realise that dreams can be fulfilled. I loved my time on the unit. I learned so much and realised that care of people with a mental illness really does not have to look like it still did in some of the old wards in the hospital; things can change, and I could be one of the vehicles of change. It was an inspiring time to be a qualified mental health nurse who believed anything is possible.

So my friend Debbi had qualified and become a registered mental nurse (RMN) and landed her first job as a staff nurse on the new child and adolescent unit. In my case, once qualified as a State Enrolled Nurse, I worked just thirty hours per week, on an elderly female ward for around two and a half years. These hours fitted in well with the care of my growing family. The three eldest children were all at school, and my marriage had ended with their father just before I qualified.

Working on this elderly female ward as a newly qualified SEN, second in command to the sister or charge nurse for around two and a half years, was a happy time. We were one big happy family even though the work was hard with forty patients, many of them incontinent and not ambulant. Working on the same ward for all that time meant that you got to know each patient really well, all their little habits, desires and behaviours. I suppose we became the nearest many of them had to a family. Not many had visitors, sadly. I sometimes took my young boys on the ward, and the patients' reaction to seeing children was quite amazing. It brought smiles, tears and also some disinterest. When sometime later I went on maternity leave to give birth to my fourth child from my new relationship, I took the baby onto the ward to show the patients and staff, and my heart melted to see their reactions. There is nothing like a new baby to melt people's hearts, but saying that, a similar reaction could be seen when anyone brought a dog or cat onto the ward, which wasn't officially allowed, but some wards adopted stray cats. Some patients loved to cuddle or stroke a baby or pet. I suppose they are not as threatening as an adult.

One of the patients used to run up and down the ward most of the day and grabbed my baby's shawl, then ran off with it! She wasn't keen to give it back either. Another lady who ran up and down all day used to regularly plonk herself down at the piano and play a very loud music hall-type song and then just stop and slam the piano lid down and run off. When I think about it now, it was a crazy environment, but we got used to it and never batted an eyelid. My older children were a little disturbed by what they witnessed and had plenty of questions!

Around this time after the end of my marriage, I had met my new partner, a nurse at the hospital, and we moved in later on together with my boys to form our own family unit. He was the scruffy long-haired man I noticed on my very first induction day at the hospital some years previously in the Afghan coat, but I never dreamt that we would become a couple years later! Strange how things turn out! So following working as a State Enrolled Nurse part-time on the elderly ward for three and a half years and eventually feeling a bit stagnant in my career, it was with his help and encouragement, even though we had a new addition to our brood of a new baby boy, that I prepared to start my training on a full-time course to become a Registered Mental Nurse, which in those days took me another two years. My second husband became the love of my life and was a father to all the children, and this man gave me the confidence I lacked and had struggled with for many years.

So as Debbi was taking up her post as a qualified staff nurse, I too was completing all my training to become a staff nurse, and my first appointment in that role was to work in the Regional Alcoholic Unit. I will come to that later. In the following chapter I feel the need to describe my memories from working in the Occupational and Industrial Therapy Units as a student nurse to gain experience and an understanding of what happened in those units.

OCCUPATIONAL AND INDUSTRIAL THERAPY

I feel it is important to mention these two experiences during my training because these areas were later abandoned in the process of change, but at the time were considered beneficial to most patients. Debbi did not work in these areas, as training experiences for student nurses changed during her time later on, and these two areas were not considered of much benefit to the training programme for nurses then.

Occupational therapy was housed in a detached modern building where multiple activities were available to all ages with different levels of mental health problems. Everything from art, crafts, cooking and life skills to talking therapy groups were available, which sounds brilliant, but the reality, due to limited resources and the willingness on the part of patients to engage, was far from brilliant. There tended to be a group of patients who loved attending and embraced many activities or kept to the things they liked obsessively. I met a female patient in the art room there who had been in the hospital a long time and never spoke. I didn't know much about her, but she could just paint wonderful caricature portraits of anyone very quickly and accurately, so that is what she did all day. I still have the one she painted of me to this day, which she signed and dated in 1976. I can't believe that she wasn't out in the world using her skills to make a good life for herself, but I didn't know her history or why she didn't talk or communicate. Hopefully someone has tried to help her.

Others did everything possible to dodge attending and would hide in bed or would go missing and wander around the grounds to kill time, swearing that they had attended when they hadn't. When asked why they didn't like going, some would say it was like going to school and felt it was patronising to an adult. Others were probably a bit lazy or felt too anxious to go. Can you imagine taking strong tranquillising medication which created feelings of numbness, tiredness and slowness, then being pushed to get busy or be positive about activities? It was an uphill struggle.

Spending time as a student nurse in the unit helped one see all these points of view, and it was also an opportunity to improve one's own craft and art skills! Many occupational therapists were in those days very keen, and I hate to say some were patronising. Occupational therapy had not always been around for some of the longer-stay patients, and some had worked in the kitchens, laundry, sewing room and gardens/farm at the hospital, but this was stopped in favour of occupational therapy because it was seen as free labour and taking advantage of ill people. Those who loved their work, having done it for years, were very traumatised by being 'sacked', as they saw it, and some became very withdrawn and relapsed. They weren't given a choice. Again the rules of the institution were paramount, and we had a long way to go before real choice was available. Those who worked in the various hospital departments felt like they had a job, were valued and were contributing to their community. Isn't that what we all aspire to?

Industrial Therapy was in a separate detached modern building and was run by laypeople with experience in factories or warehouses under the umbrella of Remploy, an organisation producing items for sale made by disabled people in a more protected environment. I think integration at work is now a more acceptable practice. So the same patients went to work Monday to Friday and earned a very small wage for their work. They had set hours, breaks for coffee and lunch, and the general aura seemed quite happy and productive. The tasks were simple and quite boring or repetitive, so chatting while working was encouraged, and it was a way of finding out quite a great deal about your fellow workers. I made purses using a hole-punching machine and packed endless amounts of hospital dressing packs (CSSD packs). I also knitted a jumper whilst sitting talking with fellow workers, which I am sure wasn't really my role, but as students we were there for six weeks, and nobody gave us any guidance or told us what to do - just observe?

Anyway, the unit was also disbanded later, as it too was seen as cheap labour and using patients for profit. More integrated working in the real world or community has been encouraged rather than within a big hospital or a protected workshop nowadays. However, I have to admit those weeks spent working in that industrial therapy unit seemed, for many, a happy, supportive environment while producing useful products. It was probably better than staring at a wall or pacing up and down locked in a ward for many years for some.

One of the most important ways to improve our mental health is to try to engage in activities that we enjoy, helping to distract us from bad feelings or enabling us to get fresh air or socialise with others. So encouragement to do that is the role of a therapist. Most occupational therapy is available in day centres, community centres or church halls in the community. The biggest hurdle is to encourage someone to get involved in something when that is the last thing they feel like doing, due to feeling anxious, paranoid or worthless. Or sometimes in life they have never engaged in any positive activity. That is probably one of the reasons why they have found themselves with severe mental health problems. I know now, living alone, that by going for a walk or joining a group activity, my mood is lifted and I feel better even though on setting out I sometimes feel, honestly, I can't be bothered. You just have to have a word with yourself and get out there!

THE ALCOHOLIC UNIT

As my friend Debbi has previously explained, she left the mainstream hospital wards on qualifying and specialised to work in a Child and Adolescent Unit. I too specialised on qualifying to work in the regional Alcoholic Unit. These units were in the same grounds as the main hospital but operated very differently and independently.

Despite us nurses having a reputation for partying and frequently drinking alcohol, it became evident to me that we were very ignorant about the effects of drinking alcohol and the damage it can do to health and society. In those days drinking was a normal part of socialising, and pubs were thriving. Although modern life has changed, the majority of the public see no harm in 'having a few too many' and are very ignorant about when that becomes a problem. When one is young, it is often felt that all the advice against any substance abuse is good but doesn't really apply to me. Having lived in France for a while, it became obvious to me that the Brits' relationship with alcohol is often unhealthy and inappropriate.

Nowadays the same applies to recreational drugs, but of course they are illegal, whereas alcohol isn't.

So I arrived to work on the Alcoholic Unit to discover that patients were assessed for suitability before admission. The main criteria being that they were at rock bottom and ready to admit they had a problem and needed to consider total abstinence, possibly forever. They were referred by their GP as part of their conditions of probation or by social workers, mainly, and assessed by the consultant from the unit.

Most patients were in a poor physical state, being physically and emotionally dependent on alcohol, so spent about a week on a general or the physical illness ward at the hospital to literally physically 'dry out' before they came to us at the unit. The drying-out process usually involved taking daily doses of high-strength vitamins and a daily reducing regime of tranquilising medication to prevent delirium tremens, hallucinations, etc. This took approximately seven days when the patient was dressed in pyjamas or nightwear, was not allowed to leave the ward and usually did a great deal of sleeping initially. They were also encouraged to start eating a healthy diet and do some exercises. Remember, these were often individuals who had 'hit the booze' hard over a long period of time, not eating or sleeping properly, and were physically showing signs of various serious illnesses. The emotional aspect is the hardest dependence to tackle, and that was the area we dealt with on the unit after the patient had 'dried out' and was no longer physically dependent on alcohol.

The first thing that hit me was that alcoholics come from all walks of life, all ages and all sexes. We had bank managers, teachers, nurses, landlords, builders and ex-prisoners. Staff and patients wore everyday clothes, and the unit was very modern with large rooms for group work, smaller ones for interviews, bedrooms, a kitchen, dining rooms, bathrooms and recreational areas. Patients were expected to attend therapy groups as required and were allowed out of the building after a few weeks but only in groups of two so they could support each other against the temptation to go to the pub or buy alcohol. This worked well on the whole, but those who occasionally went out on 'a bender' or secretly stashed alcohol in their lockers were asked to leave.

Each member of staff was a key worker to two or three patients, so could have individual sessions with them if needed, but all patients were encouraged to bring problems to the community groups to share with others and help support each other whilst living closely together during their treatment.

I learnt the skills involved in group work, art therapy sessions, and practical role-play sessions, such as going for a job interview and attending a wedding when alcohol can be pushed at you in a social setting. How to say no and what to say. Patients were introduced to Alcoholics Anonymous, and relatives were supported.

Some were offered individual sessions to help them understand their relative's treatment and to try and help them cope with their own anxiety about alcoholism. There was often misunderstanding, shame and stigma associated with the diagnosis.

One of the charge nurses gave them all a formal lecture soon after their admission about the effects of alcohol on the body. He went through every organ, and having heard that lecture myself, it was enough to scare me to death about ever drinking alcohol again. The truth is that this knowledge is soon forgotten when you are relaxed in a social setting, wanting to let go, and the drink is flowing. Which most of us have experienced during our lives and enjoyed that feeling.

We all enjoy that feeling of release from all the tensions of life, but using mind-altering substances is very bad news for some and for all of us in excess. Many are using sport, healthy eating and drinking or natural therapies and groups to find release and don't drink alcohol at all nowadays. Why does it become a problem for some, and yet others seem to manage having a drinking session now and then quite well? Yet in truth there is very strong evidence to suggest that long-term regular drinking of alcohol during your life does 'bite you in the bum' eventually as you age, contributing to some heart diseases, dementia, cancers, diabetes and other conditions. So too with overeating, lack of exercise and suffering excess stress. Nobody escapes feeling the effect of some of these factors in life unless they are perfect.

So my time on the unit was very enlightening. I loved working there, and the staff were a great team. We worked together well and supported each other. We saw many discharged after about six weeks of treatment, happy and healthy with the chance of a fresh start. Some fell by the wayside, went out drinking or fell in love and left with each other to start a new life.

One memory which sticks in my mind is the day one of our student nurses didn't arrive for work and one of our patients appeared to have left the unit, taking all his belongings. They had formed a relationship whilst she was working on the unit and had decided to run away together. She left her husband for this venture, who may have been as surprised as we all were.

The 'falling in love' between nurse/therapist and patient is quite a common thing. Feeling cared for and having someone close to listen to you, to be able to confide everything you are feeling, can be a very special thing. However, the fine line between the therapist/patient relationship and a couple's loving two-way relationship can sometimes be blurred, but it is a different thing. If a male nurse had a relationship with a female patient, he could be struck off the nursing register and lose his job, but not so for a female nurse. This rule was to protect vulnerable female patients, but surely anyone being treated for a mental health disorder is not necessarily in the best place to start a new relationship. Most certainly, feeling alone, emotionally lost and vulnerable can make one feel very attracted to a caring individual. A fact any carer working in mental health services needed to be aware of. I have often said if we could have prescribed 'unconditional love' from a suitable partner as a treatment, we would have had very high success rates!

The Alcoholic Unit's method of treatment went out of fashion, I think, or was considered dated, so other methods were tried, such as controlled drinking and treatment in the community. Of course AA still operates and addiction to alcohol is still a massive problem. I hope that we made a difference for some in those days.

LOOKING BACK

As my friend and I have both stressed, in the late seventies and early eighties, change was in the air, and new innovative ideas were being introduced or tried as the huge raft of long stay patients who had been in the hospital most of their lives were becoming elderly and had been discharged to group homes, hostels, and elderly care homes where possible, and those left were slowly dying off, sadly. Many were being cared for on elderly care wards. Most younger new admissions were being discharged after a period of treatment, back into the community. Some to their families or to flats, houses or hostels depending on their circumstances. All of it sounds quite wonderful, doesn't it, but we also know that there were and still are those who slip through the net and make up a large percentage of our homeless and prison inmates. There are all sorts of social, economical and environmental reasons for this, and there will always be exceptions to success, but it feels like we need to try a bit harder, so ongoing and better planning and understanding are always needed to make some improvement.

Alongside this change came the introduction of the Day Care Unit at the hospital, the Outpatient Department, and an increase of Community Psychiatric Nurses and Mental Health Social Workers. New units were springing up, such as the Regional Alcoholic Unit and Drug Unit, which were housed in the hospital. Also, a new Regional Adolescent Unit and Forensic Unit were opened. A Deaf Unit was also opened which would rightly concentrate on one's ability to communicate one's feelings, which are often misunderstood in the case of people with a hearing impairment.

I saw several individuals admitted to a psychiatric ward with an acute episode of a 'serious mental health breakdown', which turned out to be a misunderstanding due to inability to communicate with others, having a hearing impairment. There has been very slow progress in giving those with a hearing impairment a voice, but recently there has been much more public awareness due to the media, TV and use of celebrities. New therapies and drugs were changing approaches to mental health problems, so as newly qualified nurses, we were both in the front line of it all.

One final memory during this time is something which sticks in my mind and would just not be allowed these days, probably due to fear of litigation or breach of health and safety rules: our memorable day trips. We have both previously mentioned the feeling of 'one big happy family at the hospital', how everybody knew everybody and supported each other on the whole.

There was a great social life, drinking, dancing, partying and falling in and out of love. The hospital social club and pubs in the local town were full of hospital staff and their antics. Gossip was always rife, but not in a nasty trolling way as it is today!

Some of us frequented a local pub, especially some of the male nurses, and they knew the landlord quite well. His wife had suffered with a bipolar illness from time to time, and he knew only too well how mental health problems could affect a person and their family. He had a jar on the bar to collect money for a day trip each year to the local coast for patients who had no relatives or somehow never seemed to go out on any trips from their hospital wards. To be honest, these were often the most difficult to manage patients, in a community setting outside the hospital. That is probably why they never were chosen to go on a trip. However, we knew who they were and thought it challenging to give them a break. Something we often lived to regret!

Most long stay wards organised day trips for their patients, especially to the coast in the summer or to a famous fish and chip restaurant or to see the illuminations at Blackpool. Alternatively, there were some who were never taken out on trips, often because they could be disruptive, shout out, maybe swear or 'upset the public'. This was never said openly as such, but it was the case. Public safety and risk assessment were contributory factors.

So the nurses who were regulars at the above-mentioned pub compiled a list of 'left behind' patients, and the trip was organised. Permission must have been agreed with hospital management, but staff volunteers were sought, and yours truly stepped up to the challenge.

The coach was full, and the staff ratio was high to patients, all having volunteered on their day off. The patients who smoked were all handed a free packet of cigarettes as they entered the coach by the landlord, and all were going to have lunch and tea out during the day. It was a joy to see some of the patients' facial expressions, as they thought they were in heaven. When on their wards, they were never given a whole packet of cigarettes, as these were always handed out in ones or twos by the nurse in charge or 'keyholder', even though they had been bought with the patient's own money. This was done so they wouldn't smoke them all at once or to try to spread them out during the day. The fact is you can only smoke one at a time, and there was no consideration for the damage smoking was doing to everyone's health back then. Sadly, most long stay patients smoked heavily, as it was seen as their only comfort. Just as it was to many soldiers during the First and Second World Wars.

One guy stashed his cigarettes away and proceeded to scrounge off everyone else, as he always did, until it was brought to his attention to smoke his own – years of having nothing encouraged this behaviour, not knowing when the next cigarette was coming.

The two little old ladies who were bought a sherry each to drink with their lunch by the landlord were such a picture to behold. You could see they felt special. They were being spoilt by a tall dark stranger!

In addition, talking of drinking alcohol, we had one patient with us, a famous character at the hospital, who was like a child in a huge man's body and who downed a pint of beer in two seconds, which impressed some of the locals in the bar so much that we had to rescue him from them all buying him another and another until he projectile vomited all over the pub floor. Our nurses' mopping skills came in handy! So having drunk plenty of liquid, he decided to relieve himself all over the beautiful flower beds later, whilst we had a stroll along the promenade to take in the sea air. As I mentioned, he was a huge man, and all body parts followed suit, so several elderly ladies nearly fainted when he proudly urinated in front of them, with a big smile on his face.

The trip was hard work, but lots of fun for all, and the patients went back home tired, full of fish and chips, with memories to savour. The staff had a great time too. When I think about those trips now, I shudder about the risks involved, as nobody really took charge or claimed responsibility. It probably was an insurance nightmare, but it felt right, and we just got on with it. Nobody came to any harm apart from the public maybe, who were confronted by the 'lunatics on holiday'. Most of the staff involved were senior qualified nurses with years of experience and were pretty laid back about the whole event.

I went on several of these trips over the years, and we had to turn away many members of staff who wanted to volunteer, as the demand was huge. A really good time was had by all on the whole.

Looking back to that first day on a ward in 1973, I not only started a career in mental health nursing but also a huge journey in life over the next four and a half years when I qualified as a Registered Mental Nurse. This journey involved training in many different ways, from formal lectures in the school of nursing to moving around the hospital to work in different wards and areas, learning new things every day and experiencing a huge variety of situations and emotions. I met so many lovely people along the way. both staff and patients. Sadly a few were not so lovely, both staff and patients, but these too helped in learning and trying to understand the working of the human mind.

My memories of the years spent training were happy. I loved my job and was truly committed to every aspect of it. Also during that time my children were growing up, having graduated from the hospital nursery to school, and as my first marriage eventually came to an end, I think that was mainly because I had 'grown up', no longer the timid, very young and naive housewife and mother who depended on a husband who didn't really support us, but tended to put his own interests first. I now felt I was much more fulfilled as a person, using my brain, learning and understanding new things, feeling more appreciated by friends and patients with more confidence in myself.

It was not easy to go through divorce, but the children seemed happy to leave with me when one day I sat down and explained what was happening between their dad and me, as they had spent most of their time with me alone, while their dad was often out pursuing his own interests. He seemed very jealous of my job. Despite my trying to include him in social events at the hospital, he showed his displeasure in many ways. The final straw was when he gave me a black eye as I stood in the way of him trying to smack our youngest child. I went to work wearing dark glasses and made plans to be brave and leave him. We had survived seven years, but it was time to move on for me. I knew deep down our marriage was over and had probably been a mistake from the beginning.

It was one of the best decisions I ever made in my life, as previously mentioned some time later I formed by chance a relationship with a nurse at the hospital, who became the love of my life, and we were together for nearly 40 years till sadly his death from cancer.

Experiencing trauma in your own life can help you understand feelings of anxiety and depression, which are often the symptoms initially contributing to mental health problems to some degree. The most important thing is to be able to talk and think things through, when you are ready or able, and hopefully come out of the trauma stronger, having learned something which will help in future life. Sadly this doesn't always happen, as when hurt and angry we (humans) often find it easier to blame others and events for our problems and are unprepared to examine ourselves, share things with anyone or change our own behaviour. That is a common reason why many say therapy doesn't work for them. It is not easy to look at ourselves honestly and change. We all have various mental health self-defence mechanisms which we naturally employ to protect ourselves. However, honest self-awareness can help to produce a better person on the whole.

So by the time I had qualified, I had met the love of my life, moved in with him with my children and also met my best friend Debbi, who is writing this book with me. We worked hard and played hard. There were always plenty of parties, and the hospital had a social club where many happy hours were spent. We seemed to brush away the worries about some of the tragic stories of peoples' lives that we had dealt with in our work by having fun and living life to the full, and we certainly did that. Yet I feel we always had compassion and cared a great deal for all our patients, trying to help them as much as we could to improve their lives. The hospital was in general a happy place for many, but the time came to move on in our careers, so we went to work in the community, feeling our mass of experience would be useful in that field. It was certainly very different, as you suddenly found yourself in the patient's territory, no longer in the safety of the hospital. Predominantly you would be working alone a great deal of the time with a caseload of your own and having to make decisions as a practitioner in your own right. I was the first to branch out into the community but was later followed by Debbi, and we were fortunate to spend some years working together in the same area for several years. Our career decisions were made very separately without any consultation with each other, but we just seemed to follow very similar paths. Great minds think alike?

COMMUNITY PSYCHIATRIC NURSING - CPN

So I left the hospital to work as a community psychiatric nurse (as we were called then) in an inner city area housing as many social and emotional problems as you could mention. We were based in a local health centre as part of the general community health team and took our referrals from GPs, psychiatrists and other members of the multidisciplinary team. I suppose at that time it was pretty forward-thinking and radical. We recognised any mental health problems quickly in the community and were able to deal with them in conjunction with other disciplines easily.

Nowadays, from what I hear, things have gone backwards in that there are huge waiting times for anyone in distress to get any professional help. Most mental health workers are not as easily accessible, probably due to the fear of being flooded with referrals and being unable to cope. There are many political, social and financial reasons for this, about which I feel I could write another whole book.

During my early days as a CPN, we had a consultant psychiatrist who would come out to our office at the health centre every Tuesday morning, accompanied by a mental health social worker, and one of us nurses, usually myself, would join them to visit all the people at home who had been referred by local GPs for a psychiatrist's assessment that week. Those who had milder mental health problems would be managed by our CPN team and their GP at home or at their local health centre. These Tuesday morning visits could result in prescribing medication or therapy, admission to hospital either voluntarily or under a section of the *Mental Health Act*, or sometimes no further action, but by lunchtime around 12 individuals and their families had help and solutions to their difficulties after waiting only a few days. Obviously very serious emergency situations during the week were treated immediately by emergency services, i.e. police or ambulance, when there was a danger to life or others.

The fact that people were seen quickly and locally seemed to work very well, and I have never seen a service so efficient since. The current system these days, where you hear of people being on a long waiting list or being assessed over the phone, seems so inappropriate for anyone who is highly distressed, anxious, depressed or not sleeping often with many other symptoms. Naturally feeling scared about what is happening to them, they just want initially to be reassured and listened to by someone whom they feel they can trust and believe to have the ability to offer some help or solutions to their problems.

Our Tuesday mornings were often followed by the team lunching together after a satisfying morning's work. That particular doctor was very informal and approachable. He would often be available to us by phone to advise or suggest options and trusted us to bring patients to hospital if we felt it was needed. I fully believe that trust between colleagues, as we had, enabled our service to work efficiently, aiding our patients to get the help they needed quickly.

The consultant psychiatrist and his 'in-patient beds' at that time were borrowed from an adjacent geographical area, as there were none available within our own geographical area. However, there were some select therapies, provided in a small unit used for teaching student psychiatrists at the university, which we knew little about and had never been involved with. So in view of us being situated in a large city central area with its fair share of mental health problems, departmental change was afoot. It was interesting that historically this inner city area with a very famous teaching hospital provided care and expertise for most illnesses and conditions but had no real services for 'mental patients'. It was quite acceptable to ship those difficult patients into another area for treatment. Do I detect some stigma around this? It is true that our patients were bottom of the pile when it came to providing funds and planning new services, but things were changing.

Some time later consultant psychiatrists from the city university's medical school took over this inner city catchment area, yet they didn't liaise with us community nurses in the same manner. In fact, we knew the area well – the estates, the gangster/criminal families, the drug problems, and the severe mental health sufferers – just by working closely with people in the community for years. Sadly these 'elite' doctors did their own home visits alone and sometimes came unstuck without prior knowledge or a chaperone. This to me was a prime example of a cohesive service breaking down due to a professional hierarchy flexing its muscles and a simple lack of communication.

One such instance is when a consultant psychiatrist visited a well-known to our service manic depressive patient at home and found himself trapped in the house with an Alsatian dog who wouldn't allow him to leave, snarling at him every time he tried to stand up, while the patient escaped out the back door. He was apparently there for several hours until another family member came home. However, that particular patient had played all sorts of tricks on us nurses over the years during his manic phases, which afterwards could be very amusing, but also dangerous at times. One example was running through a medical ward and pulling out all the patients' intravenous catheters! He always needed to be sectioned and admitted to hospital when in one of these phases, which we knew and maybe could have saved the doctor having his traumatic experience.

Debbi later came to join us working in the city area, and despite the conditions being difficult at times with poverty, social problems, crime and even riots, we loved our jobs and had loads of fun, supporting each other despite mostly working alone. We carried huge walkie-talkie radios, as big as a brick, which meant we could radio in for assistance or pass on a message if needed. This was well before the use of mobile phones.

I once went to visit a young man recently discharged from hospital who had a history of serious suicide attempts. He had missed his appointments and could not be contacted at home despite several visits. He had also not been seen recently by any of his neighbours. It was quite usual to ask neighbours if they had seen someone whom we may be concerned about in those days. My instincts were that he may have harmed himself, so I radioed in, asking the police to come and gain access urgently. The police came, but also several other nurses from our team who had heard the messages on the radio. It was quite dramatic, and as the police started to batter the door open, the young man came strolling round the corner eating a bag of chips. "What the F—" he said, "but at least somebody cared about me." Better safe than sorry! On another occasion I also asked the police to gain access to a house where we found a lady who had taken an overdose, and we managed to get her an ambulance and safely to hospital, where she eventually recovered.

We continued to work in the community, running huge clinics attended by individuals who were given slow-release 'depot injections' weekly, two-weekly or monthly to control symptoms mainly of psychosis or mania. These needed close monitoring, as they could produce side effects initially, but once on a stable dose, many continued to live fairly well and symptom-free in the community for years. If people failed to attend the clinic, they would later be visited at home to check all was well, and there were those who often needed visiting at home to administer their injection, as their attendance at the clinic was irregular and their lifestyle chaotic. However, in reality the attendees at the clinic often lived alone in poor social conditions with no friends or family support. We were often the only support they had, as we kept our relationship informal and friendly so they felt able to trust us and share any problems they may have. It worked for many but was far from perfect. As a result of their illness, they were different, didn't fit in, and were often shunned by the general public, so being in the community was not always the best option, as loneliness and social isolation were massive problems.

One common situation with those who suffered from a more serious mental health problem, such as psychosis or mania, is that once on the correct medication and feeling much better after a period of being unwell, the tendency was for someone to stop taking their medication too soon without advice because they were feeling OK. Many just didn't like the way the medication made them feel - a bit slowed down or flat in mood - and younger people complained that they lost their libido or interest in anything exciting. This could lead to a relapse which could have been prevented. The longer the person remained stable, often the better the outcome, and reducing or coming off medication was more of a possibility. So monitoring medication was an important role for us nurses. Administering an injection was an easy way to know that the medication was taken, but tablets were a different story. Those with a diagnosis of mania were often prescribed a drug called lithium, and we took regular blood samples from these clients to monitor the level in their system. Too high a level could be dangerous, and no level at all could mean they were not being honest about taking any of their medication.

Some would swear they were taking their medication but were not. If people refused to take any medication, it was our role to keep in touch with them in the community to ensure they didn't relapse or become dangerously ill, namely becoming a risk to themselves or others. So I have had many conversations with someone through their letterbox while being told to 'f- off'. The importance of having a good relationship with your clients, especially when they were unwell, was vital. They needed to know that you were being honest, could be trusted and were on their side. When all efforts failed, if I was worried that someone was a risk, it was necessary to inform the doctor, and following an assessment at home by a psychiatrist and a mental health social worker, a section might be applied to admit the person to hospital. This might have involved the police gaining access to their home and was not the best way for things to go, but thankfully was fairly rare. When I heard on the news recently that a very unwell person known to mental health services had murdered three people, I asked, "How could that happen?"

Each individual was encouraged to attend some kind of daycare, but it wasn't suitable for everyone. Some only came out of their homes to get their money, a bit of food shopping, cigarettes and their injection, which may have been done all in one trip each week or fortnight. The then 'new psychiatrists' responsible for the catchment area were shocked that we community psychiatric nurses were managing a few hundred severely mentally ill people in the community with the help of their GPs and medication. "Where have they all come from?" they asked. They had been cared for by us and our 'borrowed psychiatrist' for a long time. So the process of newly assessing everybody commenced over years to the benefit of some, with a few relapses for others on the way. This was yet another example of those planning and managing a health service not communicating with those who are actually already trying to deliver it. I believe this is still happening to this day and probably contributes to some of the NHS problems we see today.

Other sides of our work then were to assess the 'worried well' who were often referred by their GP directly to us. These people often had anxiety, depression or other mental health issues which could often be 'nipped in the bud' by some talking therapy or monitoring and advice around mild medication. I honestly believe we averted many from becoming more seriously ill because they were seen quickly in a local, more normal setting. The stigma or fear associated with 'going mad' is still a very strong issue in most people's minds.

We also attended the ward rounds held at various mental health hospital units and met those who were soon to be discharged into our area, to introduce ourselves for their follow-up support at home. We were involved in teaching both nursing students on placement with us, and I presented our role to all kinds of NHS workers, including medical students at the university on request. The job was always interesting and could be different on a daily basis. We experienced riots in some of the local estates, drug dealing and violence and saw things you would never believe, but took the rough with the smooth, and our fellow workers' support was paramount.

In one particular area of 'my patch', which was renowned for drug dealing, crime, poverty and many social problems, this mix of circumstances still exists to this day, one thing feeding another, and we don't seem to have managed to break this cycle.

One day I called to see my client/patient at his maisonette. He lived with his mum, but she didn't cope well looking after him. He had learning difficulties and mental health problems which were not helped by his lack of physical care and support at home or how the local gangsters used and abused him to do their errands. That particular day he was very agitated and shaking but was unable to tell me what the reason was. I asked if he had taken his prescription medication and eventually found out he had sold it to a neighbour. I asked him which neighbour and marched along the walkway to the neighbour's house with my walkie-talkie radio on show and demanded he give me back all the medication, then proceeded to give him a lecture about taking advantage of my client and how he should be ashamed of himself. He said, "Hey, I paid good 'f—ing' money for them pills." I informed him that he had better give them back right now or he would be arrested, which he did, and explained I would be keeping an eye on him from now on and that his 'good money' was sadly spent.

I don't know what came over me, as I could have put myself in a very dangerous position, but it worked. I don't think the outcome would have been as good these days. It was over thirty years ago, and things were different. I returned the medication to my client, ensured he took what he should and spent time talking with him and his mother about better strategies to use in dealing with their problems and what help and support they could be entitled to use.

I was fortunate enough to spend an academic year at Manchester University on a Community Psychiatric Nursing course involving two placements out of the area and other shorter courses in teaching, assessing and counselling. These gave an academic basis to what I was already practising. We were living in the world of evidence-based practice, and our nurse training in the 1970s was seen as outdated, which it probably was, but it was a good basic grounding, and with plenty of hands-on experience, we learnt as we worked on the job. This reminds me of when I first started training and we had 'made up' State Enrolled Nurses in charge of wards who were promoted on experience alone and not training. The difference with us is that we continued to attend courses to expand our knowledge and were open to learning, not hiding or fearful of it, as some of them were. Every practitioner, especially in health, should keep up to date with the latest research and trends, even to question their validity sometimes. Sadly this is difficult to achieve, as someone has to continue to 'fight the war' while others are learning how to do it better or end it. Shortage of staff and lack of time make this near impossible.

Whilst on this yearly Community Psychiatric Nursing Course, the opportunity to take time out for a whole academic year in order to examine one's practice and to work in two different geographical areas, taking on a small caseload of clients with whom you could work intensely and present them as part of your studies, was a luxury but also helped you make sense of what you were doing with highly successful outcomes. Sadly, in reality, lack of funding, shortage of staff and too many referrals create less successful outcomes and very tired, demoralised staff.

I eventually left the city team, as I and my family moved house to a more rural area, and spent another 18 years or so working across that very different environment, continuing as a community psychiatric nurse, developing new skills, running psychotherapy groups and anxiety management groups, later managing the multidisciplinary mental health team and eventually becoming a nurse member of our local Primary Care Group. The changes from those early days in the 1970s were huge, and one needed to be open and embrace them, but all my past experience was so valuable, as many of the problems remained the same, and as I have said before, people's true needs when distressed don't really change much. I will recount some more of my memories as my career moved on, but my co-writer Debbi also finds herself working in the community away from the hospital environment and in the following chapter relates some of her experiences. It seems strange that our careers followed very similar paths despite no real discussion about it.

DEBBI MOVES AWAY FROM THE HOSPITAL TOO

As Angela previously experienced, I, Debbi, discovered that my next role was to take me away from hospital inpatient care forever, though I did not realise it at the time. I applied for a job with the community team for the elderly mentally ill (later to be renamed Older Persons Service, which describes the service in a more positive way). This was a 'G grade' post – promotion! My mum insisted that we should still be staff nurses and sister/charge nurses and therefore told people at home that I was now a sister!

I had succeeded and made my mum very proud. My mum's very best friend was also a nurse, midwife and Queen's nurse; we were her family also, as she had no children of her own. She too was proud but could never really get to grips with the fact I had become a mental health nurse and not a 'real' nurse! She was always keen to hear about my job and listened with great interest and respect. Both my mum and her friend were cross when I told them about the ward sister in the general hospital!

We were based in the community, in a health centre based in an inner city area renowned for having a huge ethnic minority population, social problems, poverty, drug misuse and criminal activity. This meant travelling through the city each day, which was a new experience for me, and I was not keen on it at first; everywhere was so busy! And I later discovered that I could leave my home in Wales and get to work quicker than from one side of this city to the other!

Working in the community brought a host of new experiences. Using my car every day to visit patients (who were soon to be renamed clients and later again service users), I wrote down my mileage in my battered old Austin to claim fuel payments back, which I am sure paid for most of my fuel! Haha. There had to be some return for nurses' low wages left behind again, in addition to wear and tear on our own cars.

As my friend explained, we had huge radios; they were approximately the size of a house brick and definitely did not fit in your pocket! These were two-way radios with which we were able to tell the control office where we were going in order to ensure we were safe. Along with the briefcases containing our depot drugs, I am sure we stood out like sore thumbs and attracted much more negative attention, thus making us more of a target than if we were without!

In case you are wondering what a depot injection is, it is a frequently used antipsychotic drug which is injected into the muscle, usually into the buttock but sometimes the outer thigh. (Nowadays there are newer drugs that can be given into the arm/deltoid muscle). The drugs were oil-based, and large doses were often difficult to give without a lot of pressure. The drug releases itself from the muscle over time, commonly every week, two weeks or monthly. (These are still used today, but there are also other newer drugs available nowadays).

We used to stock our briefcases with the vials of drugs, usually approximately 20, needles, syringes, cotton wool, plasters, sharps boxes, etc., and also equipment for taking blood samples from patients if necessary. As I said previously, it was obvious we were possibly carrying something of value, and this made us at risk of potential theft.

In certain areas of the patch it was a risky thing to do, and we were offered a uniformed police officer to accompany us. I recall once a brick being thrown from a block of flats! Scary, but to be honest, incidents like this were rare.

The experience of other people's lives, however, continued to amaze, interest and also sadden me. The first time I had to knock on a door terrified me! It is very different working with individuals within the safety of the hospital, but out there on your own, usually with very little information about what to expect as well, was daunting.

My first home visit (I even remember the actual address!) was not far from the office. I was due to give an injection to a gentleman with a diagnosis of schizophrenia. I was told that he was of Nigerian heritage and he was not able to speak English, but his family could. The lady who answered the door invited me in without speaking, but she smiled and ushered me through a tiny kitchen which smelled very strange.

There was a huge pan bubbling away on the cooker with a grey-coloured scum on the top. It transpired later that it was the older gent's underwear and socks being washed.

The gentleman's bed was in the living area squashed up in the corner, he was a giant of a man; he was tangled up in his bedding and did not even look as I entered the room. The lady said something in a language I could not understand, and the man turned to the wall and exposed a buttock for me to inject. This was very uncomfortable for me; not a word had passed between us, and I needed to discuss things with him. Why was he in bed? How was he managing the side effects, which were evident to me (drooling mouth, tremor, and involuntary facial movements)? I wanted to learn about his history, assess his needs, etc., but it seemed he wanted only his injection.

Not a good start! There was no way I was giving it until I at least established he was the actual patient! I managed to establish that a grandchild would be home from school later in the day, and his English was good, so I arranged to go back later, using a lot of gestures and probably lots of misunderstandings!

So I continued my visits and tried to find my way around the area without getting too lost! No sat nav then! But each member of staff was given an A-Z of Manchester, and I found it useful each evening to check my diary and plan routes which I wrote on A4 paper in large writing and left with a pencil to scribble off each line as I passed down the relevant street. However, if my radio requested me to attend an emergency mental health crisis or support a colleague… well! I was lost. But I soon learned to find my way around and discovered all the shortcuts too.

I went back to my Nigerian gentleman, and yes, his grandson was home from school. It seems his grandad had been living in London for some time with another relative, and this was how he lived. He had been very unwell in Nigeria, probably, by the description, psychotic, and his information/case notes had not followed him. The young person said that without his injection "he is crazy", so he asked me to give it to him and worry about why another day!

I did reluctantly give it to him that day, but not without being concerned; I mean, he could not even identify himself! However, the drug chart was signed and the address and DOB were correct. This was the first and definitely not the last time I had to weigh up the pros and cons of a situation and decide to take a positive risk, continuing my mantra, "If you can justify it in a court of law and it is in the best interests of the patient, then do it." It turned out that I was right to do that, as when I chased up his information, which was in transit from London, it seemed he was a very unwell and disturbed gentleman. I went to his house every two weeks for nearly 18 months, and though he smiled a couple of times, he did not change. With the exception of the smell of the pan in the kitchen, I always felt welcome, and I was rewarded with chocolates at Christmas from the family; how very kind.

Working in the community involved many challenges, not only getting lost but also making decisions alone, assessing risks alone, and learning that because you do not have the safety of the ward around you like a big blanket, you could not just walk away at 5:00pm or go away and go back to check on someone, make sure family members were ok, and even look after pets. I cannot tell you how many dogs and cats I have had in my cars, taking them to kennels, etc., whilst their owner is taken to hospital. I recall once being asked to feed a snake! I had to take a frozen mouse out of the freezer, put it in a mug of boiling water to defrost, open the lid and hold the poor thing midway into the glass tank with some tongs until the damned thing jumped up and grabbed it! Oh, it was horrible! I also had to stand on a chair to reach it, and I knocked my shins on a coffee table when I jumped down and ran away! Maybe that was the day I learned to swear!

Everyone had a great laugh in the office when I told them about it. We used to laugh a lot. I have very fond memories of our office humour; I do not believe anybody who has not done our job would understand our humour. We laughed at each other's reactions and responses to some of life's most difficult and distressing situations, but never laughed at the patients.

Someone once described it as NHS gutter humour, maybe not wrong, but I truly believe more often than not it was a coping strategy.

When I reflect on my own life and opportunities and consider the life my family are leading and compare it with some of the events I have witnessed, I often wish I could share it in detail with individuals I meet in my role today, some individuals who seem to think they are entitled to have whatever they want, whenever they want it and without working hard to get it. I was once going on a visit in a notorious block of flats in the city with the aforementioned police escort. I think he was a very new constable, and not very confident. We walked up three or four flights of concrete stairs, passing groups of youths who just stared at us (that was why escorts were recommended), then down an open walkway passing door after door. When we reached the end of the row, my patient, who was due a monthly injection, was not at home, so I left a note on a preprinted card which we were given for this purpose (well, actually, we made them ourselves). The officer commented about the smell on this walkway, and I agreed it was quite unpleasant, but sadly it was not unfamiliar to me. Another resident came towards us and asked if I was from the council, as she had reported the bad smell several times and nothing had been done about it. I agreed to follow it up. We were quickly able to identify the door which the smell came from, and we knocked and looked through the letterbox. The body of a woman (only feet visible) was on the floor inside, and there were millions of flies everywhere. I had recognised the smell of decaying human flesh from my work on the physical care ward, where some poor souls had bedsores so large you could put a fist into them. The rest I left to the young officer, who sought the appropriate help when he had stopped vomiting!

It transpired that the poor lady had died alone, and nobody had missed her for weeks. I will never forget that day, not just for the horror of it but for the fact she was so alone in the world and nobody in that high-rise block of homes had missed her or cared enough to investigate.

Another memory I have to share with you is the reverse, probably one of the saddest of my career. I was asked to go and assess an elderly gentleman whose wife had died approx. two years previously, and neighbours were concerned that he barely left the house and barely spoke when he did. The GP said the neighbours had tried knocking on the door, but although he was polite, they could not gain access. He was seen in the fish and chip shop next door, but this had reduced recently.

When I knocked on the door, he opened it with only a crack, and it took a long time to persuade him to let me in. He was an absolute gentleman, very quietly spoken and polite; his eye contact with me was minimal; he just looked at the floor, head bowed and wringing his hands. The hallway smelled musty, and he was wearing a tweed jacket and a jumper, but they were old and dusty. His trousers fell in folds over his very old slippers, which he shuffled to the side to let me in, shutting the door behind me (another rule broken… never let the door behind you be locked).

The hallway was quite dark, and I could see shapes above my head, and he slowly shuffled to another room. These shapes were moving gently and 'jingling'. I had no idea what they were until he opened the kitchen door, which let some light in.

Above my head were hundreds of metal pie holders, the sort you get from a chip shop when you buy a pie; they had been hung at different heights with pieces of sewing cotton and a drawing pin to secure them into the polystyrene tiles covering the ceiling. I really did not know what to make of it, but I was just glad to have been able to get into the house. Everything in the kitchen was covered in dust, and there was a kitchen chair close to a small coal fire which was lit but with only about three small lumps of coal. I was very careful with my questioning, as the gent was very suspicious of me. Honesty is always the best policy. I told him that I was there because people were worried about him, and he began to weep.

It soon became obvious that this gentleman was seriously depressed and undernourished and was experiencing suicidal thoughts. He had a pile of brown tablet bottles on the table which were labelled for his wife. As a CPN it is second nature to assess risk without asking questions. We look around; there is no evidence of cooking, no dirty dishes, food smells, loose and dry skin, ill-fitting clothes, poor eye contact, slow or limited response to conversation. None of these alarm bells had developed overnight. The poor man could barely speak to me, let alone express his thoughts and feelings; he did, however, nod when I asked if he would go into hospital.

Today, getting a hospital bed is very difficult, but in the 1980s, not so. I just made a call and off we went. Some of his neighbours were outside, and with his permission I quietly told them that he would be ok but he was going to hospital; one lady hugged him and said, "See you soon."

On arrival at the hospital, the usual protocols began, paperwork completed, and my gent was asked to undress and bathe. In the room were three of us (I did not want to leave him, and he seemed to want me there), another female nurse and a male auxiliary. The poor man was helped to undress without complaint, and we helped him gently, thoughtful of his dignity, but when we removed his jacket and jumper, there were another two jumpers and a shirt. The poor chap was pitifully thin; his skin hung loosely, and it was very dry. The final layer of clothing was the tatty remains of a ladies' 'liberty bodice', as they were called. I think today it would be described as a thermal vest, maybe? He was very reluctant to let it go; he whispered, "my wife's". It was put in a property bag and given to him immediately. He was bathed by the male staff, and before I left him on the ward, I noticed he already looked calmer, sitting in a comfy chair, clean and probably feeling safer.

It was after 11.00 that night before I rolled into my bed; nobody had missed me, and when I think back, lone working policies did not really exist, except for the radios! I didn't even have a colleague waiting for a quick text to say I was safe! That depressed gentleman was discharged after approx. two months, and I continued to see him at home for about a year. He had no direct family, but he and his dear wife had been very popular in the community, and they welcomed him back, continuing to offer their kindness and support.

He could never explain why he put the pie tins in the ceiling, but he did not remove them. They were actually quite pretty in a strange sort of way! He missed his wife terribly, and probably did for the rest of his life. He was a lovely man.

During 1981 the inner city area where we were based was the scene of mass protesting which lasted for two days. This became known as the Manchester riots. Racial tension and mass unemployment were thought to be the reasons, and also allegations of police officers being racially abusive and using excessive force towards black youths. I was working that day, and I and other colleagues had returned to the office at lunchtime, sensing a quiet tension in the area. We had not been in the office long when our manager told us we had to evacuate the building and leave the area as quickly as possible. My car was parked in an underground car park at the health centre; when I descended the stairs, there were youths and men, predominantly black, everywhere. I was very frightened. Most were armed with baseball bats, pieces of wood, and large tree branches. I got into my car and started to move slowly. Thankfully they let me out. "Get out of here quick," I was told, so I did! I was very grateful; maybe 10 minutes later things may have been very different, and I would not have had a car to escape in. Thankfully the motorway was much closer than the roads to north Manchester and my shared house, so I just kept driving home to Wales. I watched the news and was horrified to see the damage and the anger; a difficult and frightening time, to say the least.

Our health centre housed a pharmacy, and subsequently it was raided and badly damaged. Two days later we were back out onto those streets doing our job. Crazy but true!

Very early during my time as a community nurse, I realised I would never work on a ward again. I would like to be able to say that I enjoyed working with families, but to be honest, not many of my caseload had family, or at least had family who cared about them in any meaningful way. It seems I was destined to become a nurse who predominantly works with the more complex, vulnerable and disadvantaged individuals in our communities.

In having this role I can honestly say I have met some very strong, creative, kind, funny, and resilient people who will stay with me forever.

Schizophrenia and bipolar disorder (previously known as manic depression) were the two main diagnoses of the client group I worked with. Both are complex and multifaceted diseases.

Considering schizophrenia initially, it is such a cruel disease. As with other mental illnesses, there are various subcategories to consider, but for the sake of my memories, it is enough to remind myself that it often strikes individuals when they are just beginning their adult lives. So many times I have witnessed the devastation of young people coming back from university, being unable to cope with the course, not feeling able to mix socially, and suffering some strange and frightening experiences which they do not feel able to talk about because it is "just so weird" or "if I tell you then you will have me locked up". Probably one of the best skills a mental health nurse can develop is the ability to make the person in front of them feel safe enough to finally tell someone about their experience of, say, auditory hallucinations or visual disturbances which are so real and frightening that the person cannot believe others cannot see or hear them. Delusional beliefs, which are so real for people, no matter how unbelievable to others, are so distressing for everyone concerned. Family, friends and the community cannot see mental illness, no plastered leg or bandage, or acceptable explanation for being unwell, such as diabetes or appendicitis.

The ability to reassure and give a person hope, hope for their future, the chance of recovery, maybe even to have meaningful relationships, have a job, a decent home, everything we take for granted really.

Now, in 2025 that is possible, with the advances in science and new drugs to treat these illnesses and also a huge shift in societal attitudes to serious and enduring mental illnesses. It is still, however, a very devastating diagnosis to be given.

The early '80s brought many changes; as my friend has explained, the asylum was closing its doors and community services were growing. Being a part of moulding these services was an exciting time. We were all feeling our way; we knew basically what we wanted: never to return to the long-term incarceration of people who had done no wrong, at least willingly.

We had the opportunity to make a massive difference to people's lives, but was the community ready to embrace these people? No, it was not!

My friend mentioned loneliness; this was a very sad outcome for many. Leading lonely lives in a world where they felt they did not fit.

Try to imagine life without dreams and aspirations, or to exist without a role in life, whether it be a father or mother, a brother or sister, a shop worker or carer. Many individuals I have worked with over the years could not say what their role is in life. They could wake up in the morning (if they had been able to sleep for more than a few hours) and have no idea about how they would spend their day; it would depend on the extent of their symptoms. Not only their voices or beliefs, for example, but also what is known in services as negative symptoms.

Negative symptoms are probably best described in layman's terms in a book I have frequently recommended to students over later years (*Working with Serious Mental Illness: A Manual for Clinical Practice, Brennan, Kerr, Goldspink 2000*){5}. They describe stereotypical images which come into people's minds when considering mental illness: "maybe inexplicable and violent behaviour, as if the person is in the grip of some alien force, removed from normal life, 'mad', 'raving' 'crazed' (which of course is untrue), but they do not consider 'people who look and act numb' or people who have lost all their inner energy. They do not include the person sitting on the sofa smoking endless cigarettes and getting up only to make a cup of tea (and leaving the milk and sugar and the used teabag in a mess afterwards). Neither does it include the individual who spends two hours getting out of bed, puts on the same clothes as worn for the last week and then falls asleep in the chair an hour after getting up. Nor does it explain the families who think they no longer have any feelings for them because they hardly talk and only reply, 'Yeah, I'm ok,' in a flat and disinterested voice when asked how they are."

These symptoms have clinical terms: 'blunted affect', 'alogia', 'avolition', 'anhedonia', and 'inattention', to name a few, but this is not a lesson in understanding schizophrenia. It has taken me almost 49 years to learn what I know about this appalling illness, and I could most certainly continue to learn from the people I work alongside. Every person is different and is affected in different ways, but there are few whose experiences are anything but frightening, depressing, and confusing and often leave them feeling quite hopeless. Offering hope has always been an important part of our job.

The next chapter, written by my friend, is, in our view, an example of a venture which did offer hope. Sadly, even today the people who hold the purse strings are not people who truly understand or have even witnessed the effects of the loneliness and isolation some individuals experience when suffering from a severe and enduring mental illness. I used to believe that this was an issue because the transition from the asylum to the community left them bereft and without purpose. Sadly, today

(2025) I can still witness this sad situation much more often than I would like. However, it is a difficult balance to achieve, not creating dependency and supporting the philosophy of recovery, which is something I believe passionately about.

I will offer you an example of this for you to understand what I mean. In one of my community mental health nursing roles I started a walking group. This was not something I just plucked out of the air; I had read a great deal of research as part of my BSc (Hons) degree course, which was combined with a specialist nurse in community mental health nursing qualification. My role in an assertive outreach team at the time meant that I was working with individuals who had serious and enduring mental needs exclusively; I did not have a mixed caseload. I was also a member of a team who worked closely together, and we offered opportunities and clinical interventions such as CBT (cognitive behavioural therapy) for psychosis, family therapy and individual 1-1 sessions focussing on recovery. I can honestly say that this approach was the most effective way I have worked throughout my whole career. The emphasis on social integration developed gradually as we recognised that individuals were much more engaged when they were offered opportunities other than medication.

I mentioned a walking/photography/nature group as one example: maximum of six individuals and two members of staff. We managed to squeeze some money for waterproof coats and overtrousers, a couple of flasks for hot drinks and two rucksacks (everyone was expected to provide their own appropriate footwear) out of a friends of the local hospital fund. We used two cars and went to areas of outstanding natural beauty which were very familiar to me. The group chose the walks each week, and I do not recall anyone missing even one week for the two years we ran them. We took photos of particular areas in different seasons - snow, bluebells, autumn, etc. - and met together to share thoughts, memories and plans to do certain walks at different times. Friendships developed and there was a true sense of camaraderie and mutual support within the group.

We (the staff) deliberately avoided instigating conversations, and we were often moved by the level of support people offered each other. They spoke of medication frequently and shared feelings about their illness and the treatment; they shared frustrations, hopes and dreams, and we all laughed... a lot. We paddled in the river, lay down in the heather, listened to birdsong, identified flowers, and learned about cloud formations. I took my new puppy, and they learned about the benefits of physical contact; there's nothing quite like being able to cuddle a puppy and be licked. Can you imagine life having never experienced these things? Well, these people had not. Ever. This is probably why nobody ever missed a walk!

Sadly, it was not to continue. The small-minded managers of the day decided that it was not recovery-focussed, we should not be encouraging people to take part in something they cannot achieve independently. "These people should be doing things in their own communities," access buses (which do not travel to the middle of a wood), and go with individuals without a mental illness (they can't because they do not feel they fit). "Groups are a thing of the past; we should not encourage it" (close all support groups for stroke victims then!). You can probably tell from my tone that I was very angry about this, and although I fought really hard to defend the value of our group, the walks had to stop, but do you know what? The management did not once ask the service users what they wanted. Apparently "the NHS does not pay nurses to go wandering about in the forest on a jolly every week."

Can you imagine the management fury when I managed to get the same group of people involved in playing sports abroad! Haha, it was brilliant! The European Association for Sport and Social Integration (EASI CUP) was taking off, and we travelled to Austria, Holland and Manchester to take part in football, tennis, swimming, volleyball and bowling. Mixing with people from all over Europe who had serious and enduring mental illnesses such as schizophrenia and bipolar disorder. Much fun was had, and much chat about how to lose the large

Clozaril tummy in every language! (An unpleasant side effect of an antipsychotic drug called Clozapine). To experience flying in an aeroplane, owning a passport and being an important part of a sports team meant that memories were made which would last forever. It is OK for 'do-good service managers' to spout about scientific evidence and unacceptable practices, but they can make unforgettable and precious memories whenever they want to!

I think the original reason for telling you about this was by way of an explanation of the difficult balance between developing relationships with our patients/clients which are therapeutic but also not creating a dependency. I agree there is a very fine line, but to not be confident, to almost reach that line, is to provide a service which is not effective for the group of individuals who find being an active member of the community in which they live very challenging and often cold. Leaving the individual often sad, lonely, without purpose, and unable to build meaningful relationships.

My view of being 'paid to go on a jolly every week' was the commitment of a very hard-working, compassionate and visionary team who made a massive positive difference to the lives of people nobody else really cared about. It is strange that now in 2025 services are being actively encouraged to support service users to go out in nature, take more exercise, and meet with like-minded people! Who would have thought it, eh?!

So back now to Angela, who will tell you of a venture which we both utilised/experienced with our patients, the community asylum (our description, not theirs).

A COMMUNITY ASYLUM

Taking into account that the word 'asylum' means a safe place. There was an amazing scheme in that inner city area which needs to be mentioned because it seemed to be a tremendous success for those who had or were recovering from serious mental illnesses or were alone and unable to cope in the community.

The pressure was on to close the large institutions and discharge as many patients as possible into the community following the rehabilitation drive. Then the opening of specialised units in the hospital grounds and selling off some of the land, which later became housing estates, hypermarkets, petrol stations and restaurants, became a plan.

Also looking today at the problems we have with the homeless, prisons being full to bursting and many living lonely lives in poverty and substandard housing. Many of these individuals have mental health problems and have nowhere else to go. Society is not very tolerant, and they need asylum, somewhere safe where they are able to live supported by staff who understand them.

The above-mentioned scheme was in an inner city street, in a fairly run-down area, where this very innovative Irish lady and her husband bought a house, renovated it, then proceeded to gradually buy more houses on the street, renovating them and taking in ex-patients or individuals who needed supportive living, having experienced mental health problems.

They each had their own rooms, some shared by choice. Their meals were all cooked in one house kitchen and carried across the back street to the other houses. The houses were the smartest in the street, all comfortable, clean, well furnished and decorated. The lady owner seemed to be steering the ship, whereas her husband was kind and patient with all the residents, going to the end of the earth for them. He particularly took the elderly men under his wing and had a great relationship with them. His wife was full of compassion too and on some occasions nursed some residents at home with dignity when they reached the end of their life, providing them with their every need.

Her sister, brother-in-law and, I think, on occasions, other family members worked in various roles, cooking, cleaning and providing maintenance to the houses. The owner and her husband lived next door to the residents in their own house, but conducted all business in the house nearest to theirs. They were on call always if they were needed and never seemed to take much time off because they loved their setup. It reminded me of how life was probably many years ago in Ireland and most working class communities in England, where everyone knew and helped each other on the street. When people wandered in and out of each other's houses for a chat or to share a problem, and doors were always unlocked.

One of the community nurses in our team, also Irish as it happens, had the job of visiting the houses every week to administer any depot injections needed, to assess any resident having problems and to provide support and information to the owner and her husband. I sometimes visited them too.

We were also invited once a year to an evening party at her house, which was the best. Plenty of singing, dancing, laughing, eating and drinking in a good old Irish style.

The whole scheme was quite unique because here was a couple of kind middle-aged people who selflessly gave up most of their own time to care for and provide a home (asylum) for many who had nowhere to go and couldn't quite cope with life. Their placements in small cosy terraced houses felt homely and suited their needs. Some of the large hostels and homes that provide care don't have the same atmosphere, and staff come and go, doing their best, but are often bogged down with administration, staffing issues and poor wages, which makes them feel quite devalued.

The couple who ran this scheme were like many of the dedicated people who in later life, having brought up their own family, then take in to their homes, disabled or adults who are unable to cope living alone or even foster children often with very complex needs. I take my hat off to them! When you have led a full life and brought up your children, who eventually leave the nest, you often feel life is empty and need something to do. Often helping others brings much personal happiness, and many of us in this modern life are too busy pursuing projects to improve our own situations, not realising that satisfaction is never reached because we are never done. There is always something else to strive for. Advertising and social media make sure of that!

LEAVING THE CITY FOR ANOTHER CHALLENGE

Having moved my family to a house in a more rural area with a view to living 'the good life', growing some food and keeping some animals on a small farm, I, Angela, moved to become a community psychiatric nurse in a semi-rural area.

My husband was then a nurse manager at the hospital where we met and was responsible for a mental health unit at the local general hospital too, so he continued to work there despite our moving house and travelled further every day to work. He had been a staff nurse for many years previously, which was rare in those days, but he was always the rebel and I think made the management nervous, so wasn't considered for promotion until more open-minded or forward-thinking managers became the norm. The hospital hierarchy traditionally had been held tight by rules, traditions and even certain families, would you believe? There were stories of attending the right church or being able to play an instrument in the hospital band as a prerequisite to get you promotion in the past. Older ones amongst us can all sadly remember this kind of nepotism in large organisations in the past, when people didn't move away from their families much to find work or prior to equal opportunity laws for employment.

As previously mentioned, my husband had started at the hospital as a staff nurse on the same day as me, but we didn't know each other at the time until a few years later. He had moved from his post in another hospital in the southwest of the country, following his recent divorce from his first wife. His move north to his brother's address was to try to make a fresh start and commence working permanent night duty at the hospital. He was always very popular with staff and patients, as he had a very laid-back attitude and good sense of humour. He enjoyed a good party – a bit too much! But was kind and helpful and always supported the underdog. He was also an active shop steward in the nurses' union, which didn't always go down well with management. I know I am biased, but when older staff and attitudes retired, he was eventually offered promotion to become a charge nurse and, years later, a nursing officer. He even acted up in a senior nursing officer role for over a year because they had no replacement for someone who had left, yet when the job was advertised, they gave it to an outsider who also left after a few years for a higher promotion. So it took a long time for us to realise that we were not ambitious for ourselves but loved our jobs caring for our patients and didn't ever consider moving onwards or upwards to better things, yet there were those who did and never put down roots anywhere, just kept moving on from promotion to promotion and never really achieved much. I suppose it is a fact that people are driven differently.

Anyway, he became a nurse manager for many years towards the end of his career and, as many said, was always very approachable, continuing his laid-back attitude, as Debbi also discovered when she was in trouble on the general hospital ward and sent to be disciplined as mentioned previously.

The move for me working from within a fast-moving inner city community to a much slower semi-rural community was quite a difference. The interesting factor is that people basically are the same and their needs and anxieties are quite similar, but in those days the treatments were so different, like chalk and cheese, depending on where you lived. Nowadays, the differences in all types of health care depending on where you live, which still exist and have done for many years, are referred to as the postcode lottery. There is a great deal of work happening now to try and level things up so that all can expect the same quality of care, but a great deal depends on funding, of which we all know there is never enough. Inner cities receive more in funds due to larger populations and deprivation, but it is not always recognised that semi-rural areas have their share of poverty and deprivation, with fewer opportunities in all aspects of life, despite the views outside the windows being very picturesque!

The area I moved to had no past experience of a large mental hospital taking in those in the community who had suffered some kind of mental breakdown but instead had several 'psychiatric' wards attached to the local general hospitals, which had been established for a long time. Quite an unusual situation and a sharp contrast to the practices in the inner city university hospital mentioned previously.

This was seen as quite innovative and forward-thinking, but when you looked closely, they hadn't moved with the times for years. It was the community nurses who had been employed from other areas, with a great deal of past experience, who seemed to shake things up and introduce many new ideas.

Our manager, also fairly new to the area and having worked for many years where my co-writer and I had trained, encouraged us to be bold and, from our health centre bases, encouraged us to develop all kinds of therapies and groups for both mild to severe mental health problems, easily accessible and close to the GPs who could refer directly to us. They loved this, but the hospital management and some psychiatrists were not very happy with this. They didn't have control. Surely the patient outcomes should have been the main concern, and these were pretty good within our service. It was a great place to work and we felt we were helping people and making a difference.

We liaised with the wards, attached to the general hospitals, of which there were two in the area. Being a semi-rural area, there was often a huge distance between visits, so we were deployed in three teams to split the distances geographically and to provide us with more familiarity within a local area.

I met and worked with many who had suffered with a long-term serious mental illness for years and were very institutionalised in their behaviour yet lived mainly in the community, apart from brief periods spent in hospital when they may have deteriorated or relapsed for some reason. So in previous pages we talked about living for years in a large hospital affecting people's behaviour, yet in this area I saw similar types of institutional behaviour because the staff who looked after them seemed stuck in their attitudes (institutionalised?) and didn't work to try to change or improve the individual's life but concentrated on continuing maintenance and not taking any risks. Some of their families too seemed stuck in their lives too. It is probably a fact that things move or change much more slowly in the country than in the city or an area which attracts people from other places with more diversity.

Almost everyone in the area where they lived, or on the wards, seemed to know each other quite well and tolerated their strange behaviours at times. Maybe a rural community is more tolerant of its own? Modern-day society doesn't seem to be as tolerant. We move home to find employment and travel more, so close-knit communities become more fractured. Also modern pressures don't have much room for being tolerant, because everyone seems to be under pressure and is busy trying to look after 'number one' in difficult times. Or is it that we are all trapped into striving to better ourselves, achieving perfection or expecting too much?

Anyway, in this rural area, there seemed to be more extended families living closer to each other, so a support network could be easily available, but surprisingly enough, some had never even visited another town or village in the area and had all kinds of suspicious or negative beliefs about people in those places. So coming from an inner city area, it was a shock to me to see so many old narrow attitudes about life. Perhaps one of the major facts behind this is that there were fewer opportunities to join varied activities or pursue varied and interesting careers. Many young people needed to leave the area to 'get on in life'.

With all the above in mind, it made a difference to how you could help people with mental health problems to get back on track with their lives after a breakdown, as resources were limited. There was daycare, but it was fairly blocked with the same people attending for many years and not moving on. As community nurses, we again ran community clinics to administer depot injections in health centres and encouraged attendees to have a chat and a cup of tea in a group situation. The conversation was light and open, asking what they had been doing during the week. Talking about current news and asking their opinions was a way to get a conversation started. One conversation which comes to mind was about the national lottery, which was a fairly new thing at the time. I asked if anyone had ever bought a ticket and what they would do if they won a million pounds. This proved to be an interesting question, as someone came up with "I would take a week's holiday in Blackpool if I won." What was evident is that many could afford a week's holiday in Blackpool and didn't need a million pounds to do that, but they believed that it was such a big luxurious thing to do that they could never arrange it or do it. In general their aspirations in life were very limited indeed. They just had no idea or comprehension of what could be available to them if they won a million pounds. Years of lack of confidence, education or encouragement, in addition to feelings of anxiety and other symptoms associated with a long-term mental health problem, contributed to their above view of the world and their life in it.

We worked taking referrals of patients from their GPs, who may have been displaying symptoms of anxiety or depression for all sorts of reasons. Some were individuals who were suffering with grief, which is not a mental health problem but a normal reaction to a life event. When does grief become abnormal? How does someone get through losing someone in a violent act or terrible accident? How do you come to terms with the loss of a child? Watching a loved one become victim to a terrible illness with no chance of recovery is devastating.

All these examples came my way, who presented as very distressed individuals initially coming to see their family doctor seeking help because they couldn't sleep, had no appetite, felt anxious all the time, low in mood or just couldn't get on with their lives and were terrified that they were going mad. Many other strange beliefs and symptoms were evident too. A family doctor can be a good listener and prescribe mild medication to help such individuals, but they just haven't got the time to give to such individuals, of whom there are many, ourselves included, probably at some time in our lives. So I was one of a team of three nurses based in a health centre, and we took referrals directly from the community health team in addition to those referrals from the psychiatric hospitals following discharge, supporting those living in the community with more severe mental health illnesses.

The 'worried well', or those who, as mentioned above, visited their GP in a desperate state, often as a last resort because they didn't know where to turn, were asked if they would be happy to come to an appointment with a community nurse who was experienced in understanding the types of symptoms they were experiencing. If the word 'psychiatric' was used, it would often put the fear of God in most people, to be honest, or they would become very defensive and say, "There is nothing wrong with my mind."

In truth the types of situations that came my way were, for example, a mother whose son was killed in a car accident. He was one of three passengers who died, and the driver survived. They were all teenagers and were driving too fast round a bend. This had happened over six months ago, and she was unable to sleep and had been unable to cry or admit how angry she felt with the driver. She had never been in her son's bedroom since it happened, and her relationship with her husband was in tatters because he didn't know how to help her.

She was very uncommunicative and defensive, but by gently letting her know that you were trying to understand how awful she was feeling, being there for her, encouraging her to talk about her son, what he was like and what had happened, and also by asking the right questions, she started to express her feelings, and in time she cried – a lot. After just three sessions she started to grieve and move on and was able to sleep and communicate more with her husband. She would never get over losing her son so young but was able to find a way to carry on and live with her grief. Sadly, so many are unable to deal with the death of a loved one, but our reaction to losing someone close is a painful but normal situation and we can be helped in time to pick up our lives and carry on.

Another type of loss is when a partner leaves you. A young man was referred from his GP who couldn't sleep because his wife had moved out with their young son to her mother's house, saying she needed a break. She couldn't give him a reason, and he was devastated because he didn't know what he had done wrong. It was obvious he was very devoted and sensitive and found it difficult to consider his own needs, rather than the needs of others. When I asked if he had considered that she may have met somebody else, he couldn't entertain that as a possibility. Sadly for him, as it turned out that was the case, and after two sessions of talking about it, he was able to move on, accepting she had left and that he hadn't necessarily done anything wrong. He was still able to see his son regularly and think about his own life and options open to him in the future.

Those 'affairs of the heart' can make us all feel pretty desperate, and the terrible feelings we experience when someone we love rejects us are quite normal and sometimes we need the support or listening ear of someone we trust to get through. We don't really need the help of a professional in such normal situations, but if there is nobody there to help, these feelings can become serious and destroy one's confidence or mental well-being.

Another example of the type of worried well who came my way is of an active grandma who panicked whilst babysitting her grandchildren. They were asleep in bed, and her son and his wife were out at a social event for a few hours. She became so anxious that she rang her son to come home as quickly as possible. It took a while for her to tell him in tears that she suddenly became terrified that she would harm the children in some way and could not be trusted. This was totally irrational to him, as she had always been a capable grandparent, but it turned out that she had been suffering from anxiety for several months, which had become worse, and she was unable to control it. When I saw her, she was very ashamed about her thoughts, but they were very real to her. Through a few sessions asking her about her life, it became evident that she had had a whole load of stress to deal with in her life and had taken this for granted. Learning to be self-aware about anxiety and how to care for oneself using relaxation as a strategy helped her enormously, and she began to feel more confident and happier with herself. She accepted she wasn't going mad, losing control or capable of harming anyone against her will.

Anxiety, as we know, is a fight-or-flight response within us all, but when this becomes excessive for no apparent reason, then some form of help early on can turn our life around to become a more mentally healthy individual. As a result, we taught anxiety management strategies both individually and in groups running for eight weeks at a time at the health centre with very positive results.

The other kind of groups we conducted were psychotherapy groups, which were quite in vogue at the time, and our manager at the time was a big fan. The individuals who were invited to these groups and selected to attend were many who were often well known to the local psychiatric services, often diagnosed as having a personality disorder or someone who never seemed to be able to move on in life, wearing their 'mental illness badge' as an excuse for everything that didn't go well. It sounds brutal, but the group setting allowed fellow members to challenge and share feelings whilst supporting each other to find new ways to get on. The role of the therapists, usually two of us, was to say very little but guide and ensure that things were fair and individuals felt supported. It could become quite hostile at times, or there could be long periods of silence which were difficult for some, but the workings of a group can be very interesting and powerful. Fellow group members can be very honest about others' faults and also very supportive by sharing similar feelings. The reality TV programmes which have become so popular nowadays remind me of the power of group psychotherapy, as they, in their groups trying to live and function together for a while, sometimes in difficult circumstances, can stir up all kinds of emotions. They nearly all, following their experience, when interviewed, say that they learned a great deal about themselves and were greatly affected by the experience. We all find ourselves in all sorts of groups during life which hopefully help us form who we are and our ability to function in society. Maybe not being exposed to many group situations in life can cause us some difficulty with our own identity and mental health?

So the other work of assessing new referrals and supporting those with severe mental illnesses living in the community was a large part of our role. Also, working in a community health centre, we were able to teach many of the other disciplines who worked there about mental health problems and often went out on joint visits with district nurses, health visitors and social workers.

As Debbi has already mentioned, a change of management came, and so, with no consultation, did our practice. So we were removed from health centres and based in new mental health resource centres at a considerable cost, the reasons being that we were supposedly spending too much time with the worried well and the more severely mentally ill were being neglected. New drugs were available and new therapies called psychosocial interventions were being proposed. As we have continually mentioned in this book, change is always on the horizon as time moves on, especially in healthcare. I presume change happens based on research for better outcomes or to help fill gaps in care to the benefit of patients/clients. Having been in the service so long, I sometimes wonder, as in mental health services, if we seem to go round in circles and have often followed trendy fads which can burn out very quickly.

In times gone by we used to bleed people to make them better. We also used leeches as a treatment for some illnesses. In psychiatry we gave people electric shocks, put them in insulin-induced comas and cut some tissue in brains to reduce severe anxiety. It all sounds very barbaric but did have some scientific backing and seemed to work for some. The importance of continued research resulting in change and acceptance must be supported.

I honestly believe now that our interventions with the worried well worked well and prevented a great many problems becoming worse. Counselling services were developed to fill that gap, but they seem overstretched with long waiting lists and sometimes became overwhelmed because often their training and experience were limited. Patient/client views and outcomes will reveal whether this is true.

The Mental Health Resource Centre has now been closed, and I think Mental Health Services are based in teams in a more specialised service, so you need to be referred and assessed before seeing anyone, and of course there are long waiting lists.

The current preoccupation with Mental Health or lack of it, does seem to be about trying to cope with everyday stresses in a world where we don't put up with things as we did in the past, are less tolerant and have much higher expectations of life. We are faced with prejudice, racism, bullying and abuse, which have always been there but don't seem to lessen despite our awareness.

The ability to cope and be more mentally healthy can surely come with education, starting with small children and continuing throughout their education and experiences both at school and at home. Learning to be able to talk and share when feeling sad or upset. Learning how to deal with bullying and how to say no when you really don't want to do something. Also learning to be kind and tolerant and trying to understand that being different is OK.

This all sounds idealistic in a perfect world, which we don't have, but there are many schemes, groups and initiatives around which are trying to tackle many of the above. However, from modern media sources, we are sadly learning about the alarming number of children experiencing mental health problems and being diagnosed with ADHD or autism, which is putting huge pressure on the already stretched Child and Adolescent Services.

What are the answers? What is the way forward? Are we becoming a society who are obsessed with needing perfection and need a label for everything? What is normal?

I couldn't answer these questions, but I can have an opinion, and maybe going back to the real needs of people, which I have mentioned before, such as shelter, warmth and nourishment in a physical sense and feeling loved, having friends and having some meaningful occupation in a psychological sense, would be a start to promoting good mental health. Sounds a bit basic, but if every parent and teacher could provide this to every child, it would be a great start. Finally, instilling and teaching good values are imperative to a cohesive, caring society.

Good luck with all that!

FURTHER REFLECTIONS AS BOTH TOOK OUR DIFFERENT PATHS

I would like to wind up some of my ramblings with some thoughts about where this book came from and why myself and my good friend felt it would possibly be a good idea to write this memoir. We were very touched in our lives by our experiences and felt others starting off a career in mental health services may learn and be touched by these accounts. The general public too may be interested in the topic and the historical changes which have taken place. The sad and funny stories bear witness to many of these too.

As Debbi has previously stated, I have often been asked, "How could you do that job?", "Were you frightened by some patients exhibiting disturbed behaviour?" The answer is yes, sometimes we are all frightened by violence or fear for our own safety, but in all the years I worked in the job, I can only recount a few incidents when I felt threatened or uneasy.

For example, I was walking through one of the wards at the local hospital and discovered several staff grappling on the floor with a very angry young man who was making all kinds of threats and who had been chucking furniture around the ward in a dangerous manner. The charge nurse threw the medicine keys at me and asked me to draw up a prescribed injection in the clinic and help them administer it to the young man who was not going to calm down any time soon. I was known to the staff and trusted them to know that this needed to be done, so helped them out. After some time the young man started to calm down and was escorted to a 'time out room' to sleep and calm himself with the help of the medication. On the way to the room, he proceeded to spit at me and tell me he would find out where I lived and kill my family. It was some months later when I was walking down the corridor of the hospital that I saw him rushing towards me and braced myself to be greeted with a smile, a hug and the news that he was much better and being discharged tomorrow, and how was I doing? He had obviously forgotten or forgiven me for that injection, much to my relief, so I proceeded to have a normal positive conversation with him.

Another time while visiting a young woman in the community, I felt the need to alert the doctor to ask for a home visit with a view to a compulsory admission to hospital by section, as she had become very disturbed, shouting, dangerously smoking, threatening her elderly mother who was terrified and refusing to open the door to anyone offering help.

Sadly she had a diagnosis of multiple sclerosis and had been prescribed some steroid medication to aid reduction of inflammation, which in some rare cases can cause a psychotic breakdown. I knew the young woman and had had a good relationship with her, but despite there being a note on her records to say do not prescribe steroids, as she had already had an episode of psychosis before, someone had not read this and prescribed them for a deterioration in her mobility caused by the MS.

So she had, as previously, become very paranoid and disturbed. She was totally out of character and threatened to report me to all the authorities for gross misconduct if I asked the doctor to visit and would not let me in the house. Her elderly mother was imprisoned in the kitchen. So after being admitted to hospital again on a section, being treated with the right medication and some months later being well enough to go home, we resumed our good relationship and she apologised to me for all she said to me, having remembered her threats.

These examples demonstrate how, when mentally unwell, a person doesn't behave as they would normally and, if left untreated, can become quite dangerous, and it is not always personal who they choose to harm. Just sometimes a case of being in the wrong place at the wrong time.

The guy who arrived at the main city train station in his pyjamas to go to London to collect his earldom from Buckingham Palace whilst in a manic phase of his illness was stopped by the railway police due to his strange behaviour and was eventually arrested as he became very irritated and aggressive. I was contacted to help, and when hearing his name, knowing him well, I went to the station. He was in a cell, handcuffed and very agitated, being guarded by two large policemen. When I arrived, the man recognising me said, "Thank god you are here, darling; these idiots are totally out of line. I need to get to London. Do you have a fag? I am gasping, darling." I sat on the bench with him and provided him with a cigarette and encouraged him to tell me all about what had happened. He became less irritable and aggressive but had no insight into how inappropriate his behaviour had been. He was loud and garrulous, skipping quickly from one topic to another. He had not been sleeping and had no time to eat or rest. Later he was assessed from the doorway by a timid doctor and social worker who didn't get too close, as he was a large, intimidating man, resulting in him being admitted to hospital on a section of the *Mental Health Act*, about which he was not very pleased, so he was manhandled into a van whilst fighting and verbally aggressive on the way.

This particular guy was not normally a nasty person. He was a well-educated, well-mannered man when well, but sadly had a diagnosis of manic depression and had suffered a relapse. The nature of this condition usually presents itself with a person not sleeping, becoming agitated, irritable, unable to think calmly, behaving and spending money erratically and easily becoming angry. The other side to mania is that the person can become very amusing and cheeky and take risks, which can be very dangerous too.

Having a relationship with someone throughout their well and unwell periods helps in being able to convince them that maybe they need to take various measures to remain stable and prevent admissions to hospital. The person needs to trust you and your advice, which doesn't always happen, but we needed to keep trying, visiting despite the response.

Another lady, one of my clients with the same diagnosis, had a large family and was a great mother, wife and grandmother, but when she started to become unwell, she would always fall out with someone, not sleep well and become chaotic in her life. The family members knew to ring up and would say, "She is going off again; please help." She was always friendly to me when I visited, but if she was becoming unwell, she would open the door, tut, walk off and say, "What do you want?" It took many skills to convince her that she needed help, but with the family's help we often managed to turn things back to normality. Taking regular medication was a key feature too, as often when you are in a manic phase, you feel euphoric and don't have time or feel you don't need medication.

So the question about being frightened doing my job with those who may be rude or aggressive whilst suffering a mental health problem is that these individuals are not in control of their feelings and emotions and are not behaving this way by choice, so need some help. They often have a story to tell and have been coping with untold stress, worrying alone for a long time. These are often the ones who care for others at the expense of themselves or have no self-worth or confidence. On the other hand, there are many out there in the world who choose to be rude and aggressive for their own ends, and these are the real ones to be frightened of. In other words, don't be frightened of the mad ones, but be wary of the so-called sane ones!

So my good friend Angela and I found ourselves touched by what we learnt and saw in our careers, and yes, perhaps we needed to be a certain kind of personality to do the job. Dare I say a little mad or unconventional ourselves? Maybe it was a 'calling' after all, which we were very unaware of in the early days of our career. All I know for sure is that we met and formed relationships with some lovely people, both staff and patients, along the way. My co-writer and I have a special bond and will always be there for each other, I am sure. We are busy with our own lives and families, especially grandchildren these days, whom we love dearly, but can pick up the phone any time to share our own news, thoughts or problems and trust the supportive response we are bound to get no matter what. You can't ask for anything more than that, can you?

When Angela and I started this memoir, it came from within ourselves, from the realisation that each time we met or chatted on the phone, it was always about the same thing… our memories of our time in the asylum and how proud we are to have been a part of the massive changes mental health services have seen. Quite surprisingly, as it has developed, we realise that although the changes were enormous, and individuals are no longer incarcerated behind the high walls and forgotten about, there are few people we can share our true beliefs with. This is the part of our work which began the process but appears to have taken a second place in the development of this memoir. Friendship. I am sure there are many groups of individuals who can claim to have long-lasting and important friendships which have developed in the workplace with like-minded people; it is inevitable, I guess, to share with people who truly understand. To experience, witness, and be part of working in the asylum during the time we were there is an example of this type of friendship. It feels almost cathartic to talk of those times. Sometimes, it was actually quite disturbing to witness some of the cruelty and the suffering, but to deal with those experiences (which at the time were just 'all in a day's work'), it needs to be shared with someone who truly understands without having to use words sometimes. Also we witnessed and were often party to times when the level of understanding, care and even a demonstration of loving kindness prevailed in the most complex of situations. Mental health nursing is not a job that finishes at 7:00am or 5:00pm. It is a role that continues until you have done what you can in any circumstance. That has been my experience, though I have to say the same rule does not appear to be the case consistently today, but mental illness and care have changed dramatically. As I have said previously, science has excelled and treatments have improved, and the extreme distress often witnessed in the earlier days of our careers is not often seen (thank goodness). Therefore the recovery model begins at first contact nowadays.

Please don't misunderstand me; there were so many positive experiences in the workplace and many, many fun times. I briefly mentioned earlier about the 'NHS gutter humour'; we laughed so much when on and off duty. We socialised a lot. Despite the long 12-hour shifts and persistent need for overtime to make ends meet, we went out a lot. Pubs, occasionally clubs or live music gigs, but predominantly the hospital social club. Suffice to say it was rife with relationships, affairs, and many friendships. Too much alcohol was consumed regularly, and the use of cannabis was commonplace. I do not recall conversations focussing on the hospital, though. Probably because we would be back on duty within a few hours anyway!

Angela and her husband had children, so they were her priority, along with her beloved husband and wonderful friend to me, but as a family they were always welcoming, and their home was always open, so I made full use of that. I was often to be found sleeping over on one of their large squashy sofas with their dog, and mine, surrounded by noise, bickering, wrestling fights, huge pans of food and lots of love. When I had my own family, I so often used their parenting styles. I was so positively influenced by their open, honest, fearless way they brought up their large family, and I have watched in awe over the years how well they have all done in life.

When they moved away I missed them all terribly. Thinking back towards the end of my time in the big city, I was quite homesick; a relationship with a guy who worked at the hospital had ended, and I started to go home more often, seeking support from my friends who had returned from university/college and were now working nearer home. I met a man from home, or should I say a relationship developed with a man from home whom I knew, and I wanted to be at home more, or him with me, in the city. I went on holiday with Angela and the gang to France, and my love (boyfriend at the time) joined us for a week (very brave!).

We had hired a minibus for the two weeks for us all to go to France. I decided I would go alone to the airport to pick him up and take him back to the gîte where we were all staying. It was a huge bus with a sunroof and no power steering! I gave myself plenty of time to get there, obviously wanting to make a good impression and not be flustered. As I approached the car park, a storm broke and the heavens opened. I drove straight through a height restriction and virtually removed the sunroof! Well, I was flustered then! Police arrived with weapons and very bad-tempered faces. I was told to go to another car park outside the airport after I had answered many, many questions and signed forms, etc., all in French. I hadn't a clue what I was doing! Then I ran to the airport in the rain. My dress was stuck to my body like a skin, and my hair was dripping! The rain stopped just in time for my future husband to stroll out of the airport into the sunshine looking very handsome and cool, haha! Great start!

It was during this time in France that I knew my career path was changing. I wanted to go home, settle down and have my own family, but that was a scary prospect. I was so happy where I was, but I missed my pal and her family when she moved out of the inner city team to a more rural area. Another big issue was my dog! My dog sitters had reduced in numbers when they moved, and I could not leave her while doing a 12-hour shift; she would have to go home, and if she did, then so would I.

I thought at the time that my work life could never be the same if I went back to the rural area I came from; my training and my work as a community nurse in a city would be different in a rural area, with a very different demographic and pace of life. The people I had met, my friends, and the systems I worked within were so familiar and safe. I had learned my way around, and to be honest, I believed I was a good nurse and felt I had a lot to offer the community I worked in. However, I was beginning to feel preoccupied with thoughts of being at home. I was fed up with missing phone calls or waiting for letters from my 'boyfriend' (feels strange calling him that when we have been married for 40 years!) up and down the motorway in a battered old car which had a strange but funny malfunction. If I drove below 55-60 miles an hour, the cassette music I was playing would slow down; as I picked up speed, it would return to normal! Strange but true.

We bought our first home together for the princely sum of £17,000, a fortune in those days! I lived there whilst waiting for our wedding day and travelled every day back to the city to work. I did this for approximately a year, and though it was hard, at least I went home every night. There was an unspoken understanding that we were living together before we were married, but one day my dad phoned the house for something in the morning, and my husband-to-be answered the call! I thought Dad would go nuts! But he merely suggested that this should not happen because if my grandfather had called, it would be a different story and he would be very disappointed. How much things have changed!

I couldn't find work in the community close to home, as these teams had not yet developed, so I worked in a hospital for individuals with learning disabilities and mental illness. It was a small asylum basically. In the countryside in a beautiful old building which was definitely haunted, I quite honestly thought that I did see a ghost there one evening on a late shift; strangely, I was not frightened at all, and the staff who had worked there for many, many years, confirmed this as a genuine 'sighting'.

It was a very different role from what I was used to, but I enjoyed it very much. There were lots of opportunities to make changes, but like going back to the big hospital, many staff were very reluctant to try new things. These were the 'made up' SENs, staff who had nursed for a very long time but without formal qualifications. The majority worked hard and did care, but as in most institutions, there were the odd few who resented my presence and efforts to do things differently. I believe it was the beginning of opportunities for people who had lived in the hospital for many years. Myself and other staff with a vision took a group on a short holiday to Blackpool. This was an event which was organised by a couple who closed their establishment and opened it to hospitals like ours. The individuals we took all had new clothes to go (not from the hospital bundles), new shoes, the works! All from Marks and Spencer's!

We had a wonderful, memorable time, including walking along in the pouring rain, seeing the sea (for the first time for one lady) and having to get out of the hotel at 3:00am due to a fire alarm! Not funny at all, especially as one gentleman was totally immobile, and he was also a large chap to get out of bed into his wheelchair! Thankfully it was a false alarm, but scary just the same!

The day of my wedding dawned at the same time as a community mental health team was developed locally and I was successful in my application. So I left my job to be married and start a new, more familiar job. I was thrilled to see some of the ladies from the hospital outside church before I went in, all clutching lucky heather, picked from the hospital grounds and wrapped in tin foil. We halted proceedings for a short time whilst chairs were made available for them to come in and sit down and watch my marriage. What a lovely day. Of course my wonderful friends were there to celebrate with us.

It was then so much changed. My writing buddy and her husband left the UK to start another chapter of their lives together, both retiring from their jobs as mental health nurses. I knew I would miss them, but we kept in touch. Nothing would ever end our special friendship; it merely changed shape.

I am convinced that it was our experiences in the asylum that brought us together. It is impossible to explain what it was like, each day being different and each experience having the opportunity to stir so many emotions within you. Much of it remained unspoken, but in the company of like-minded people, you did not need to find the words; we knew that we understood.

My worries about my job being different were put to rest when I went on a joint visit with a mental health social worker.

We met at the house and introduced ourselves, had a brief conversation about the referral and walked up the path of a well-kempt garden to the front door of a bungalow on a housing estate. Thick white net curtains were on the window next to me, and my colleague knocked on the door. Next thing I knew, we were both holding on to each other as a huge Alsatian dog was snarling and drooling and making every effort to get through the glass to eat us! We had both encountered dogs, but trust me, this was scary! I am actually laughing now as I am recalling it. A lady opened the door and apologised about the dog and said it was safe in the kitchen, and we could go into the lounge (the room the dog had left). We pushed each other through the door, neither of us wanting to go first. I was doing my best not to laugh nervously. We accepted the offer of a cup of tea and were left alone in the lounge whilst she went to make it. When she closed the door securely behind her, we both noticed claw marks gouged into the back of the door from the very top to the bottom; this was a huge beast for sure! We sat gingerly on the sofa, and then my colleague pointed to a large bone on the rug by the fire, nudged me with his elbow, and said, "That is the remains of the last community nurse that came here!" How I managed to continue with the assessment when the lady came back I have no idea, but assess her we did. This is a good example of our professionalism; it really was a memorable event, one of those that you had to be there to appreciate it, but I know the lady had no idea that we had been laughing.

That takes me back to the humour and the relationships we build within the role of treating mental illness. That moment helped me to realise that it was no different over the border, and I quickly felt safe and knew I was going to be a part of another team with high standards, clinical excellence, and the ability to support each other through the remarkable journey our careers were on. I remain friends with that social worker today, and we have both met and become friends with many others too.

So, my next chapter began; my life was good, we were happily married, and we soon had our first of two wonderful sons, and our second came along three and a half years later. We are very proud of both of them, and it seems my dedication to my career did not have a detrimental effect on them, as they both are leading good lives. I would not have managed without family to help, particularly my parents-in-law, who helped with childcare so much.

My job was just as interesting and challenging. But my priorities changed; juggling being a nurse, wife and mother was difficult but worth it.

Mental health services were on the brink of a huge change again, and I was lucky enough to be in the thick of it. 1983 brought the new *Mental Health Act*{2} and community care was developing quickly. As if I didn't have enough to think about, I embarked on a degree, BSc (Hons) and specialist Community Nurse for Mental Health qualification, and because I had diploma credits, I did this in one year. I was then able to really forge ahead with my career, finally retiring in 2024 after almost 50 years in clinical practice.

I decided to leave the narration of my journey after myself and Angela went our separate ways, as this was a journey we were on together, and though my journey continued for many years, it was the time we were touched by madness that we wanted to highlight, and for my part, I believe we have done that. Yet in other ways it inevitably led to a big question for me regarding current practice: are all these individuals today really Mentally Ill? Why do we always have to put a label on feelings and normal life experiences and differing ways to cope with these experiences? That is a question for someone else maybe, but despite improvements in our knowledge, understanding and treatment options available, serious and enduring mental health difficulties exist still today, but again, I am sad to say, these individuals struggle to receive the full treatment they would benefit from because the NHS is short of funding and Mental Illness is again left wanting in the funding stream. Also, the label of Mental Illness has been given to individuals who, in my view, are not mentally ill, but are individuals who have not learned, for many reasons, how to cope with some of the difficulties life throws at us.

CONCLUSION

Throughout these pages we have talked a great deal about mental health and mental illnesses, the experiences we had, the things we saw, the things we learned and the way we felt during those years. We have mentioned briefly about our training to become nurses and how we were very proud to become qualified in the end. We never started out to become nurses but stayed with that career, loving it most of the time and gaining much from our varied experiences.

I feel it is a must to dwell a little on the plight of nursing. In the 1970s and 1980s we were constantly taught that we were not considered to be a profession because our training was not university-based. So we were considered skilled manual workers, and our pay definitely reflected that. Nurses' pay was very low in the 1970s, and I remember there being much unrest, a few strikes and sitting down on the main road outside the hospital in protest with others to stop the traffic and cause disruption to fight for better pay. We were moved on by the police and managed to get our pictures in the local paper. These protests were happening up and down the country then, and we did eventually get *The Salmon Report (1966)*{6}, which looked at reviewing nurse management and nurses' pay. I remember this did result in, as we thought then, a large increase in our wages, but till this very day nurses have been left behind, worked hard and felt unappreciated.

Nowadays training to become a nurse is university-based, but most seem to feel they don't have enough time to fit everything in, such as practical training, studying, trying to make ends meet and having a life. Many leave because they can't cope with it all. I hear that the current students don't always get enough practical experience on the job, so feel nervous when they have to do certain procedures on a live patient. I hear too that many qualified nurses are still poor and have to use food banks or can't ever consider buying a house.

Why do we treat nurses this way? Nursing was considered a 'vocation', not for everyone but for those who enjoyed caring for others. We can understand that, but nurses still have to eat and live somewhere and are entitled to have a family if they want. This all costs money, and despite gaining promotion, I can reflect that we always struggled financially and certainly discouraged our children from becoming nurses because we felt it was a great deal of hard work for little reward. The powers that be need to realise that we all need to look after our nurses. They are the backbone of the health service, and with others, they all got us through the pandemic, working tirelessly, and continue to care for us in many different situations. Oh hang on, we did stand outside our houses every Thursday and clap.

Both Debbi and I are avid readers, more so now we are retired, and regarding nursing, I was taken aback to read this written by a nurse, Vera Brittain (1933){7}, who worked during the First World War: *"The nursing profession is considered so holy that its organisers forget that nurses are just human beings with human failings and human needs. Its regulations and values are so Victorian that we even have to do our work in fancy dress, struggling perpetually with an exasperating seven-piece uniform, always changing caps, collars, aprons and waist belts that accumulate germs."* Thankfully things have changed a great deal today, but we experienced all the above in our careers, as we mentioned previously. Plus, she goes on to say that calling nursing a vocation is its worst handicap, allowing irresponsible authority to be left free to indulge in a type of exploitation excused by its habitual camouflage as 'discipline'. Again we experienced rules and practices in our careers which were about keeping nurses subservient, in their place and grateful. Hopefully things have changed. Despite all this we loved our jobs and wanted to tell you all about it.

We hope that you have enjoyed reading this memoir as much as we have enjoyed writing it. From starting our training 'by default' we never dreamed that we would be so influenced by what we saw and heard over many years within different experiences. We hope our readers gain some knowledge or understanding about how mental health breakdown can affect all of us in life, but our main aim was to consolidate our very similar thoughts and feelings around how we were significantly TOUCHED BY MADNESS.

GLOSSARY

AA	Alcoholics Anonymous
AA	Automobile Association
Auxiliary	A nursing assistant with no formal nursing qualifications supervised by a nurse
Charge Nurse	The male equivalent of a nursing Sister
Community Nurse	A nurse who works solely in the local community
CSSD pack	Sterile hospital dressing pack used to treat and cover wounds
Made up SEN	A nursing assistant with many years' experience, who was awarded a State Enrolled Nurse qualification in the past, as there was a shortage of qualified nurses at the time
Matron	The head of all nurses in the hospital
Nursing Officer	A nurse manager governing a group of wards or units in the hospital
RMN	Registered Mental Nurse working in mental health care
SEN	State Enrolled Nurse
Sister	Female nurse in charge of a ward or unit
SRN	State Registered Nurse working in physical care
Queen's Nurse	A nurse who has been recognised for their commitment to high standards of care and leadership.

REFERENCES

{1} Mental Health Act (1959).

{2} Mental Health Act (1983).

{3} Lunacy Act (1890).

{4} Mental Health Act (1930).

{5} Brennan, John, Robert Kerr, and Sarah Goldspink, *Working with Serious Mental Illness: A Manual for Clinical Practice* (London: Bailliere Tindall, 2000).

{6} Salmon, Brian. *Salmon Report on Senior Nursing Staff Structure* (1966).

{7} Brittain, Vera, *Testament of Youth* (London: Victor Gollancz, 1933)